The Barretts Oesophagus Mastery Bible: Your Blueprint for Complete Barretts Oesophagus Management

Dr. Ankita Kashyap and Prof. Krishna N. Sharma

Published by Virtued Press, 2023.

While every precaution has been taken in the preparation of this book, the publisher assumes no responsibility for errors or omissions, or for damages resulting from the use of the information contained herein.

THE BARRETTS OESOPHAGUS MASTERY BIBLE: YOUR BLUEPRINT FOR COMPLETE BARRETTS OESOPHAGUS MANAGEMENT

First edition. December 29, 2023.

Copyright © 2023 Dr. Ankita Kashyap and Prof. Krishna N. Sharma.

ISBN: 979-8223987406

Written by Dr. Ankita Kashyap and Prof. Krishna N. Sharma.

Table of Contents

DISCLAIMER

The information provided in this book is intended for general informational purposes only. The content is not meant to substitute professional medical advice, diagnosis, or treatment. Always consult with a qualified healthcare provider before making any changes to your management plan or healthcare regimen.

While every effort has been made to ensure the accuracy and completeness of the information presented, the author and publisher do not assume any responsibility for errors, omissions, or potential misinterpretations of the content. Individual responses to management strategies may vary, and what works for one person might not be suitable for another.

The book does not endorse any specific medical treatments, products, or services. Readers are encouraged to seek guidance from their healthcare providers to determine the most appropriate approaches for their unique medical conditions and needs.

Any external links or resources provided in the book are for convenience and informational purposes only. The author and publisher do not have control over the content or availability of these external sources and do not endorse or guarantee the accuracy of such information. Readers are advised to exercise caution and use their judgment when applying the information provided in this book to their own situations. The author and publisher disclaim any liability for any direct, indirect, consequential, or other damages arising from the use of this book and its content.

By reading and using this book, readers acknowledge and accept the limitations and inherent risks associated with implementing the strategies, recommendations, and information contained herein. It is always recommended to consult a qualified healthcare professional for personalized medical advice and care.

Introduction

"Opportunity often arises in the midst of struggle." — Albert Einstein We learn a fact from the perceptive intellect of Einstein that is particularly meaningful to people dealing with Barrett's oesophagus complications. It is more than simply a situation; it is a challenge that begs for an answer and a chance for change. Are you prepared to take control of your health and go on a journey? Barrett's Oesophagus is a complex esophageal lining disorder that frequently leaves patients feeling scared and confused. What if, however, I informed you that the map to navigating this maze is contained within this book? I, Dr. Ankita Kashyap, have devoted my life to the integration of holistic health and medical science. With my team, I've created a handbook that goes beyond conventional management, providing a variety of food programmes, lifestyle adjustments, and self-care techniques designed to empower and calm you. Turning the pages will reveal a knowledge haven, with every chapter serving as an ally in your pursuit of wellbeing. The tactics in this book are not just therapeutic suggestions; they are the keys to opening the door to a fulfilling and peaceful life. Have you ever considered options for your treatment beyond anxiety and medicine? It's time to enter a world where your illness doesn't define you but instead opens doors to reveal hidden strengths. What if you had access to the very techniques that could change your health? The question remains, "How far are you willing to go for dominion over Barrett's Oesophagus?" just when the route appears to be obvious. You'll find out in due course, but are you ready for the revelations that lie ahead?

"In the middle of difficulty lies opportunity." - Albert Einstein

The words of Albert Einstein resound deeply as we approach the study and management of Barrett's oesophagus. This disorder, which is frequently veiled in medical jargon, presents as a challenge that can change one's life as well as a physiological change. However, this issue also presents a huge chance to take control of one's health and transform what could otherwise appear like a dire situation into a monument to human tenacity and resourcefulness.

Einstein's knowledge has unprecedented relevance for people who manage Barrett's Oesophagus in a tight space. It is an invitation to rise beyond the constraints placed on one by a diagnosis and look for the bright side that could very well lead to a more fulfilling existence. This book serves as your guide through the frequently choppy waters of this condition.

There are a lot of unanswered problems and worries regarding Barrett's Oesophagus, which is defined by the aberrant alteration of the esophageal lining. Here, in the midst of ambiguity, widespread notions about the illness are called into question. One could be misled by the dominant narrative to think that their destiny is predetermined by the vagaries of their illness. Is that really the case, though?

I, Dr. Ankita Kashyap, am here to present an alternative viewpoint and a comprehensive strategy for treating Barrett's oesophagus. My team and I have discovered numerous tactics that go beyond standard medical care through thorough research and practical practise. This book serves as an invitation to go into the unexplored fields of nutritional intervention, psychological toughness, and lifestyle change.

The insights presented here are the result of years of research supported by data, not just theoretical musings. They are offered with the hope of offering practical, workable solutions. This is your manual for comprehending the subtleties of the illness, learning how to live with it, and eventually becoming an expert in its treatment.

With an open heart and a sympathetic touch, my reader, I am creating this cerebral connection with you. These pages have been brought to life by your insatiable curiosity and will to take charge of your own health. Let me pique your curiosity and lead you through instances in which the concepts of holistic health turn the impractical into the feasible.

Imagine a world in which your daily regimen protects your body from the harsh effects of Barrett's oesophagus, your meals serve as a barrier rather than merely food, and your resolve keeps your mind from being overwhelmed with anxiety. This book seeks to shed light on this pathway, not simply a possibility.

The winds of change whisper a question to you as you stand on the brink of discovery: how will your tale play out from here? A piece of the puzzle will fit together with each chapter, unveiling a blueprint for comprehensive Barrett's Oesophagus management. A plan that can be altered, modified, and tailored to your particular path.

Are you ready to embrace the tactics and realisations that have the potential to completely transform your life and take this leap of faith? Your mastery blueprint is right in front of you; all you need to do is take the initial step toward change.

Thus, I'm extending an invitation to you to turn the page, immerse yourself in the knowledge that lies ahead, and journey with me toward total Barrett's oesophagus control. Come with me on this voyage, as the discoveries that lie ahead will undoubtedly spur action, inspire hope, and ignite a deep metamorphosis. Open the mastery bible to get your blueprint.

Understanding Barrett's Oesophagus

Defining Barrett's Oesophagus

It is essential to comprehend the jargon related to Barrett's Oesophagus in order to interact with the material in this book. Understanding the key terms is essential as we delve into the intricacies of this ailment and the extensive management techniques. With this knowledge, we can start to sort out the complexities surrounding Barrett's oesophagus and open the door to proactive health management and well-informed decision-making.

In order to begin this process of learning, it is necessary to create a concise and well-structured glossary of terms that are necessary to understand Barrett's oesophagus and how it is managed. We shall define the following terminology so that everyone has a clear understanding:

1. Barrett's Oesophagus
2. Gastroesophageal Reflux Disease (GERD)
3. Dysplasia
4. Endoscopy
5. Metaplasia
6. Esophagus
7. Biopsy
8. Adenocarcinoma
9. Dysphagia
10. Proton Pump Inhibitors (PPIs)

1. Barrett's Oesophagus:

Barrett's Oesophagus is a disorder marked by the atypical conversion of the lower esophageal mucosa into tissue resembling the intestinal lining. Long-term exposure to stomach acid, frequently as a result of gastroesophageal reflux illness, is the main cause of this change (GERD). Barrett's Oesophagus is a serious condition since it is linked to a higher risk of esophageal cancer.

It's easy to compare understanding Barrett's Oesophagus to the idea of a garden whose scenery shifts with time. Barrett's Oesophagus causes a change in the esophageal lining, which reflects the effects of outside influences and the body's adaptive reaction. This is comparable to changes in plant development and soil composition.

2. Gastroesophageal Reflux Disease (GERD):

The chronic illness known as GERD is characterised by reflux of stomach acid into the oesophagus, which causes inflammation and discomfort. In addition to causing symptoms like regurgitation and heartburn, reflux can hasten the onset of Barrett's oesophagus if treatment is not received.

The experience of a river spilling its banks during a storm can be compared to visualising GERD. Like the irritation and inflammation associated with GERD, the reflux of stomach acid into the oesophagus causes anguish and changes the normal landscape, much like the surge of water beyond the river's bounds.

3. Dysplasia:

The term "dysplasia" describes aberrant cell proliferation, which is frequently seen in relation to Barrett's oesophagus. It is a serious issue since it may worsen into a more severe type of aberrant cell growth, which raises the possibility of developing esophageal cancer.

Comprehending dysplasia is analogous to identifying an error in a building's architectural blueprint. Dysplasia is a divergence from normal cellular growth patterns and, like design defects, can cause structural instability. If left untreated, dysplasia can cause severe difficulties.

4. Endoscopy:

Endoscopy is a diagnostic process that involves visualising the internal anatomy of the stomach, duodenum, and oesophagus using a flexible tube equipped with a light and camera. It is an essential tool for determining the degree of damage and tracking Barrett's Oesophagus development.

The idea of using cutting-edge technology to explore unexplored areas is analogous to the endoscopic procedure. Barrett's Oesophagus can be better understood by endoscopy, which makes it possible to see and evaluate the inside geography of the digestive system, much like an expedition uses advanced equipment to unearth hidden regions.

5. Metaplasia:

Metaplasia is the term used to describe the change from one type of cell to another. This is frequently seen in Barrett's Oesophagus, where columnar cells replace the usual squamous cells in the oesophagus.

The modification of a habitat to meet the requirements of a different species is analogous to the idea of metaplasia. Metaplasia denotes a shift in cellular composition, reflecting the body's adaptive reaction to outside stimuli, just as an ecosystem may change to make room for new organisms.

6. Esophagus:

Food and liquids can more easily travel through the oesophagus, a muscular tube that joins the neck and stomach for processing. It is crucial to the digestive process and maintaining its health is vital to general wellbeing.

Knowing the function of an oesophagus is similar to realising the importance of a bridge in joining two different places. The role that the oesophagus plays in carrying food emphasises its importance in the body's physiological functions, much like a bridge facilitates movement and communication.

7. Biopsy:

During a biopsy, a tiny sample of tissue is taken out and examined under a microscope to check for abnormal cells, such as those that could indicate dysplasia or malignant alterations in Barrett's oesophagus.

The idea of a biopsy is comparable to the forensic science procedure known as investigative analysis. Similar to how forensic specialists meticulously gather and analyse evidence to reveal important details, a biopsy allows medical personnel to closely study tissue samples, providing insight into the cellular makeup and possible anomalies inside the oesophagus lining.

8. Adenocarcinoma:

Barrett's Oesophagus cells can give rise to adenocarcinoma, a form of cancer that poses a serious risk to those who already have the disorder.

It is similar to identifying the appearance of an invading species in an environment to comprehend adenocarcinoma. The emergence of adenocarcinoma signifies the incursion of cancerous cells into the oesophagus environment, requiring close observation and treatment, much like the entrance of alien species can upset the equilibrium of an ecosystem.

9. Dysphagia:

Dysphagia, a symptom usually associated with Barrett's Oesophagus, is difficulty or discomfort when swallowing. It can arise from anatomical alterations or inflammation in the oesophagus.

Dysphagia is similar to running into a barrier on a well-traveled route. Dysphagia emphasises the influence of esophageal alterations on swallowing function by acting as a barrier to the normal passage of food and fluids, just like an obstruction obstructs traffic flow.

10. Proton Pump Inhibitors (PPIs):

PPIs, or proton pump inhibitors, are drugs that lessen the production of stomach acid. They are often administered to treat GERD symptoms and lower the risk of Barrett's oesophagus damage caused by acid reflux.

PPIs work in a manner similar to that of a regulator regulating a river's flow. Just like a regulator controls the amount of water to avoid flooding, PPIs control the amount of acid produced in the stomach, reducing the negative consequences of acid reflux and aiding in the treatment of Barrett's oesophagus.

Conclusion:

We have uncovered the complexities of Barrett's Oesophagus and its significance in the context of holistic health care through our investigation of the terminology related to the ailment. We have prepared the basis for a thorough understanding of Barrett's Oesophagus and created the framework for the in-depth investigation of its management options in the upcoming chapters by clarifying these essential terms and demonstrating their linkages to practical ideas.

The Anatomy of the Oesophagus

The oesophagus, commonly referred to as the food pipe, is a muscular tube that is essential to the digestive system of humans. This essential structure makes it easier for food and liquids to go from the mouth to the stomach, which starts the digestive process. Comprehending the complex structure and operational principles of the oesophagus is essential for appreciating the consequences of Barrett's Oesophagus and devising efficacious interventions. We will examine the intricate construction and operation of the oesophagus in this chapter, as well as how Barrett's Oesophagus impairs normal physiology.

The oesophagus connects the throat to the stomach and is around 25 cm long. It moves through a variety of anatomical structures and interacts with the tissues and organs in the neck, chest, and belly. The oesophagus is composed of multiple structural layers that facilitate its mechanical and physiological activities.

The Outer Layer:

A layer of connective tissue called the adventitia covers the outside of the oesophagus and serves to attach it to surrounding structures, preserving its location within the body and offering structural support. Additionally, during swallowing and peristalsis—the coordinated muscle contractions that drive food through the digestive tract—the adventitia helps the oesophagus move and move more easily.

The Muscular Layer:

The muscular layer of the oesophagus, which is made up of smooth muscle fibres arranged in an outside longitudinal and inner circular orientation, is located beneath the adventitia. The peristaltic action, which is necessary for moving food from the mouth to the stomach, is made possible by this muscle arrangement. These muscle fibres contract and relax in unison to propel food in a sequential manner that promotes effective digestion and absorption of nutrients.

The Mucosal Layer:

The mucosa, the innermost layer of the oesophagus, is in direct contact with food and liquids that are swallowed. Stratified squamous epithelium, a specialised tissue that guards against chemical and mechanical harm, lines the mucosa. The oesophagus needs to be protected from the stomach's acidic environment and the abrasive quality of food items by this protective epithelium layer.

Barrett's Oesophagus and its Impact:

The typical architecture and cellular makeup of the oesophageal mucosa experience major changes in the context of Barrett's oesophagus, resulting in a condition called metaplasia. The hallmark transition is the replacement of the intestinal lining-like columnar epithelium with the protective squamous epithelium. The primary cause of this metaplastic alteration in the oesophagus is the prolonged exposure to stomach acid and bile reflux, which is a defining feature of gastroesophageal reflux disease (GERD).

The Metaplastic Transformation:

Barrett's esophageal metaplastic transformation is a significant cause for concern because it is linked to a higher risk of esophageal cancer called adenocarcinoma. The oesophagus becomes more vulnerable to dysplastic alterations and cellular abnormalities when squamous epithelium is replaced by columnar epithelium, increasing the risk of malignant transformation. The important effects of Barrett's Oesophagus on the structural integrity and functional dynamics of the oesophagus are highlighted by this change in cellular composition.

Functional Implications:

In addition to causing anatomical changes, Barrett's oesophagus can interfere with the oesophagus's regular physiological processes. The oesophageal mucosa's protective layer is compromised by the metaplastic alterations, making it more vulnerable to harm from mechanical trauma and acid reflux. This vulnerability makes symptoms like dysphagia, regurgitation, and heartburn more persistent and lowers the quality of life for those with Barrett's oesophagus.

The Role of Inflammation:

Chronic inflammation of the oesophageal mucosa is another characteristic of Barrett's oesophagus in addition to the metaplastic alterations. Prolonged exposure to bile and stomach acid causes tissue irritation and immune cell recruitment, which in turn triggers an inflammatory response. The persistent inflammatory environment exacerbates the cellular abnormalities and further erodes the oesophagus's structural and functional integrity, adding to the complexity of Barrett's oesophagus.

Data and Facts:

Based on epidemiological research, the prevalence of Barrett's oesophagus is thought to be between one and two percent in the general population. This condition's prevalence highlights the importance of comprehending the anatomical and physiological changes linked to it, as well as the critical requirement for all-encompassing management approaches to reduce the likelihood of the disease developing worse.

Furthermore, statistical studies have shown that people who have Barrett's oesophagus have a markedly increased risk of esophageal cancer; in fact, the relative risk is thought to be between 30 and 40 times higher than in the general population. These striking findings highlight how crucial it is to clarify the anatomical and functional ramifications of Barrett's oesophagus in order to support proactive health management and well-informed decision-making.

The nomenclature used to describe Barrett's Oesophagus pathophysiology and oesophageal anatomy can be complex and difficult to understand. The reader's grasp of the intricate anatomical and physiological dynamics at play will be improved by simplifying and breaking down the complex phrases and concepts to aid in comprehension.

Key Takeaways:

To sum up, the oesophagus plays a crucial role in the human digestive system by acting as a passageway for food and liquids to reach the stomach. Understanding the impact of Barrett's Oesophagus requires a solid understanding of the complex anatomical and functional anatomy of the oesophagus. The normal physiological activities of the oesophagus are disrupted by the metaplastic alterations and chronic inflammation typical of Barrett's oesophagus. This highlights the important need for comprehensive care measures to reduce the risk of disease development and related consequences.

For proactive health management and well-informed decision-making, a thorough grasp of the anatomical and physiological changes is crucial as we negotiate the complexity of Barrett's Oesophagus and its consequences for oesophageal health. The following chapters will cover the detailed management approaches for Barrett's oesophagus, incorporating the fundamental understanding of oesophageal anatomy and function to enhance clinical results and patient care.

Risk Factors and Causes

Creating a thorough management plan for Barrett's oesophagus requires a thorough understanding of the risk factors and causes of the condition. We can empower people to make educated lifestyle and healthcare decisions to reduce their chance of having this condition by recognising and clarifying these factors.

1. Gastroesophageal Reflux Disease (GERD)
2. Family History and Genetic Predisposition
3. Obesity and Excess Body Weight
4. Tobacco Use and Smoking
5. Dietary Factors and Nutrition
6. Age and Gender Disparities
7. Chronic Gastric Helicobacter pylori Infection

a. One of the main risk factors for Barrett's oesophagus is GERD, which is defined by the reflux of stomach contents into the oesophagus. Barrett's Oesophagus develops as a result of the oesophageal mucosa's metaplastic alterations brought on by prolonged exposure to acidic stomach contents and bile reflux.

b. There is a clear correlation between Barrett's oesophagus and GERD, as clinical research has shown. People with persistent GERD have a markedly increased risk of acquiring this ailment.

c. Effective management and treatment options are essential for people with GERD in order to reduce the risk of Barrett's oesophagus. To relieve the symptoms and lessen the chance that the condition may advance, doctors may advise lifestyle changes, medication, and, in certain situations, surgical procedures.

a. An higher chance of acquiring Barrett's Oesophagus or esophageal cancer is associated with a family history of the disorder. Hereditary factors and genetic predisposition are important variables in Barrett's oesophagus susceptibility.

b. The genetic basis of Barrett's oesophagus has been highlighted by the identification of particular gene variants and polymorphisms linked to an increased risk of the disorder through genetic investigations.

c. People who have a family history of Barrett's oesophagus should be routinely screened and monitored for any early indications of metaplastic alterations. This will allow for proactive management and intervention to reduce the likelihood that the disease will advance.

a. There exists a substantial correlation between obesity, namely central adiposity, and a higher likelihood of developing Barrett's Oesophagus. The pathophysiological reasons behind this illness are partly explained by the metabolic changes linked to high body weight.

b. The influence of obesity on oesophageal health has been highlighted by epidemiological studies that have demonstrated a strong correlation between the prevalence of Barrett's oesophagus and obesity.

c. Among people who are overweight, weight management techniques—such as dietary adjustments, increased physical activity, and behavioural therapies—are crucial for lowering the risk of Barrett's oesophagus.

a. Tobacco smoke contains carcinogens that cause harm to the mucosa lining the oesophagus, making people more vulnerable to Barrett's oesophagus and its sequelae.

b. Persistent exposure to tobacco smoke causes oxidative stress and cellular damage, which in turn contributes to the metaplastic alterations seen in Barrett's oesophagus..

c. In order to lower the risk of Barrett's oesophagus and mitigate the negative health impacts of tobacco usage, smoking cessation therapies and programmes are essential.

a. Eating acidic and spicy meals might make GERD symptoms worse and may even hasten the development of Barrett's oesophagus.

b. The integrity of the oesophageal mucosa may be compromised by inadequate dietary intake of specific nutrients, such as dietary fibre and antioxidants, making the mucosa more susceptible to metaplastic alterations.

c. Barrett's oesophagus must be managed with nutritional counselling and dietary changes, such as avoiding trigger foods and encouraging a balanced diet full of necessary nutrients.

a. Barrett's esophagitis is more common as people age, with those over 50 having a larger risk of developing the illness.

b. Barrett's oesophagus disproportionately affects men, with a higher prevalence seen in communities of men.

c. For the purpose of facilitating early detection and intervention, age-appropriate screening and surveillance for Barrett's oesophagus are crucial, particularly in older adults.

a. Barrett's oesophagus may become more likely if there is a persistent infection with Helicobacter pylori, a bacterium linked to gastritis and stomach ulcers. This is because the bacteria can exacerbate the inflammatory environment in the oesophageal mucosa.

b. Individuals may be more susceptible to metaplastic transformations due to cellular alterations in the oesophageal mucosa brought on by the chronic immunological response that Helicobacter pylori infection triggers.

c. When necessary, the removal of Helicobacter pylori infection may be taken into account as a prophylactic strategy to lower the risk of Barrett's oesophagus, particularly in people with a history of chronic gastritis or stomach ulcers.

It is clear from navigating the complex web of risk factors and causes related to Barrett's oesophagus that a thorough grasp of these components is necessary to develop efficient management plans and advance oesophageal health. The diagnostic modalities and screening procedures for Barrett's oesophagus will be covered in detail in the following chapter, which will also clarify the critical significance that early detection plays in maximising patient care and clinical results.

The third chapter, "Diagnostic Modalities and Screening Protocols," of Barrett's Oesophagus Mastery Bible: Your Blueprint for Complete Barrett's Oesophagus Management, is available now..

Signs and Symptoms to Watch For

For Barrett's Oesophagus to be managed pro-actively and treated early, it is imperative to recognise its symptoms. By clarifying these signs, people will be better equipped to seek care when they need it and make educated decisions about their healthcare, which will improve their general health and quality of life.

1. Persistent Heartburn and Acid Reflux
2. Difficulty or Painful Swallowing (Dysphagia)
3. Unexplained Weight Loss
4. Chronic Cough and Hoarseness
5. Bleeding or Anemia
6. Chest Pain and Discomfort
7. Esophageal Strictures and Narrowing

a. One of the main signs of Barrett's oesophagus is persistent heartburn, which is frequently accompanied by reflux of acidic stomach contents. The development of this illness is aided by the mucosal irritation and inflammation caused by the prolonged exposure of the oesophageal mucosa to stomach reflux.

b. Heartburn and regurgitation are common symptoms of stomach acid reflux into the oesophagus, which sets off a series of inflammatory reactions that require careful monitoring and treatment.

c. Clinical studies have repeatedly linked acid reflux and chronic heartburn to Barrett's oesophagus development, which emphasises how important it is to identify and treat these symptoms as soon as possible.

d. In order to identify the underlying cause of persistent heartburn and develop focused interventions to reduce symptoms and stop the disease from getting worse, a thorough examination by medical professionals is necessary for those suffering from the condition.

a. Dysphagia, a condition marked by difficulty or pain during swallowing, may indicate that Barrett's Oesophagus is progressing to more severe stages, such as dysplasia or cancer. Swallowing becomes difficult as a result of the structural alterations in the oesophageal lining that jeopardise its functional integrity.

b. Barrett's Oesophagus dysphagia signals the need for thorough evaluation and monitoring in order to identify possible problems and direct the most suitable course of treatment.

c. Clinical observations have demonstrated the importance of dysphagia as a vital symptom requiring immediate medical evaluation, establishing it as a key clinical feature in the advanced stages of Barrett's Oesophagus.

d. People who have trouble swallowing or are in pain when doing so should have comprehensive diagnostic tests performed, such as endoscopic exams and imaging studies, to determine the degree of oesophageal involvement and enable focused therapies.

a. Unexpected weight loss, especially when Barrett's oesophagus is involved, can indicate problems or severe disease. Therefore, a thorough evaluation is necessary to identify the underlying causes and develop effective therapy plans.

b. The metabolic changes linked to advanced Barrett's Oesophagus, such as malnutrition brought on by dysphagia and metabolic disturbances, are responsible for inexplicable weight loss and emphasise the importance of routine clinical assessment.

c. Unexpected weight loss has been linked to advanced Barrett's Oesophagus stages in clinical investigations, which highlights the significance of identifying this symptom as a possible predictor of the disease's course.

d. To promote optimal nutritional status and overall well-being, individuals experiencing unexplained weight loss in the context of Barrett's Oesophagus should undergo thorough nutritional assessments and clinical examinations. This will help identify and address the underlying contributory causes.

a. As a result of refluxate aspirating into the larynx and respiratory passages, persistent reflux of stomach contents into the oesophagus may cause respiratory symptoms, such as persistent coughing and hoarseness.

b. Barrett's Oesophagus extra-esophageal symptoms, like persistent cough and hoarseness, require interdisciplinary assessment by otolaryngologists and gastroenterologists to determine the degree of oesophageal involvement and to direct focused therapy.

c. Clinical studies have shown that Barrett's Oesophagus, chronic cough, and hoarseness are related, emphasising the necessity of thorough evaluation to treat these extra-esophageal symptoms.

d. Patients who have a persistent cough and hoarseness should be evaluated thoroughly by medical specialists, who should perform laryngoscopic examinations and reflux monitoring in order to determine the degree of extra-esophageal involvement and to enable customised therapies.

a. Barrett's Oesophagus mucosal erosions and ulcers may make people more vulnerable to gastrointestinal bleeding, which can manifest as melena or hematemesis with anaemic symptoms.

b. Periodic bleeding in Barrett's oesophagus signals the need for immediate medical care and endoscopic assessment in order to locate the bleeding source and start the necessary treatments.

c. The clinical literature has extensively demonstrated the correlation between Barrett's Oesophagus and gastrointestinal bleeding, underscoring the importance of identifying and managing these hemorrhagic consequences.

d. When someone exhibits symptoms of anaemia or gastrointestinal bleeding, they should be evaluated by a physician as soon as possible. An endoscopic examination can help determine the cause of the bleeding and manage it so that any problems can be avoided and timely action can be made.

a. Chest pain and discomfort associated with Barrett's oesophagus may be caused by abnormal interactions between the oesophagus and surrounding cardiac structures. Therefore, a thorough evaluation is necessary to distinguish between cardiac and gastroesophageal etiologies.

b. In order to clarify the underlying mechanisms and direct specific therapeutic methods, the examination of chest pain in the setting of Barrett's oesophagus requires a multidisciplinary approach including gastroenterologists and cardiologists.

c. Clinical studies have shown how common chest pain and discomfort are in people with Barrett's oesophagus, highlighting the necessity of a thorough assessment to treat these clinical manifestations.

d. Patients presenting with pain and discomfort in the chest should have comprehensive cardiac and gastrointestinal assessments in order to distinguish between esophageal and cardiac causes and to enable the development of suitable treatment plans.

a. The development of luminal narrowing and fibrotic strictures, which are signs of more advanced Barrett's Oesophagus, can cause dysphagia and make it difficult to pass food and liquids.

b. To relieve dysphagia and enhance the oesophagus's functional integrity, endoscopic examination and dilatation treatments are required in cases of esophageal strictures and luminal narrowing.

c. Clinical evaluations have shown a link between Barrett's oesophagus and the emergence of esophageal strictures, emphasising the necessity of focused therapies and endoscopic monitoring to treat luminal constriction.

d. Endoscopic evaluations and dilation operations should be performed on patients exhibiting dysphagia and luminal constriction in order to relieve strictures and enhance esophageal patency, which will enhance swallowing efficiency and dietary intake.

It is clear from navigating the complex landscape of Barrett's Oesophagus signs and symptoms that a thorough grasp of these clinical manifestations is essential to encouraging early discovery, proactive management, and the best possible patient care. The next chapter will cover Barrett's oesophagus surveillance tactics and diagnostic modalities, emphasising how important early detection is to improving patient outcomes and clinical results.

The Barrett's Oesophagus Mastery Bible: Chapter 3 of Your Blueprint for Complete Barrett's Oesophagus Management, "Diagnostic Modalities and Surveillance Strategies," is the next chapter.

Diagnosis: Procedures and Tests

This chapter's main goal is to give an overview of the diagnostic techniques and tests that are frequently employed to identify Barrett's oesophagus. It also provides a thorough understanding of the clinical investigations that are necessary for an accurate diagnosis and subsequent management of this condition.

Assembling the necessary tools, such as biopsy forceps, endoscopic equipment, histopathological processing facilities, and the knowledge of qualified medical professionals who are adept at carrying out and interpreting diagnostic procedures, is essential before starting the diagnostic process for Barrett's oesophagus.

Barrett's oesophagus is diagnosed using a variety of modalities, from preliminary screening tests to confirmation diagnostic procedures. All of these methods contribute to the overall evaluation of oesophageal mucosal alterations and the detection of dysplastic or neoplastic abnormalities. The diagnostic evaluation roadmap is a series of steps that advance from non-invasive screening instruments to invasive endoscopic procedures, and ends with histological characterization to determine the existence and severity of Barrett's oesophagus.

1. a. i. In order to determine the frequency and duration of oesophageal acid exposure, ambulatory pH monitoring is a useful non-invasive technique that can help diagnose the pathological acid reflux that is specific to Barrett's Oesophagus.

ii. By inserting a pH probe into the distal oesophagus, it is possible to continuously monitor pH values for a duration of 24 to 48 hours. This allows for the identification of instances of aberrant acid exposure and the correlation of these findings with clinical presentations.

iii. When diagnosing and treating patients who may have Barrett's oesophagus, the examination of data from ambulatory pH monitoring systems provide vital information on the existence and intensity of gastroesophageal reflux.

b. i. In order to test the motility and functional integrity of the oesophageal musculature and to help diagnose dysmotility disorders and esophageal sphincter dysfunction linked to Barrett's oesophagus, esophageal manometry is a vital non-invasive technique..

ii. Intraluminal pressures can be measured by inserting a pressure-sensitive catheter into the oesophagus. This allows for the assessment of peristaltic function and the detection of any underlying motor disorders.

iii. The interpretation of the results of esophageal manometry contributes to the complete evaluation of Barrett's oesophagus and helps to guide the diagnosis of motility problems by providing important information about esophageal peristalsis and sphincter function.

2. a. i. The primary diagnostic procedure for Barrett's oesophagus is upper gastrointestinal endoscopy, which allows for direct imaging of the oesophageal mucosa and the identification of distinctive mucosal abnormalities linked to the disease.

ii. By directly visualising the mucosal lining of the oesophagus through the insertion of a flexible endoscope, Barrett's Oesophagus-related dysplastic or metaplastic changes can be more easily seen.

iii. Targeted biopsies are taken during endoscopy from suspected regions of the distal oesophagus, yielding histopathological specimens necessary for a conclusive diagnosis and risk assessment.

iv. Follow-up care for patients with proven Barrett's oesophagus entails routine endoscopic assessments to monitor the development of dysplastic alterations and the course of the disease, which in turn informs future management plans.

b. i. The diagnostic yield of routine endoscopic exams is increased by the adjunctive use of chromoendoscopy or virtual chromoendoscopy techniques, which improve mucosal characterisation and the identification of minute mucosal anomalies suggestive of Barrett's oesophagus.

ii. By adding EUS to the diagnostic toolkit, patients with suspected or confirmed Barrett's oesophagus can evaluate the layers of the oesophagus and local lymph nodes, which can provide important staging information.

3. a. i. The goal of the histopathological analysis of esophageal biopsies is to identify the distinctive histological alterations that are suggestive of Barrett's oesophagus and to validate the existence of columnar metaplasia with intestinal characteristics.

ii. Histopathological grading of dysplastic alterations within the metaplastic epithelium serves as a reference for risk assessment and treatment selection, making it easier to identify high-risk patients who require more stringent surveillance or life-saving measures.

a. Detailed diagnostic evaluation and the development of complete management plans require the integration of diagnostic results with clinical presentations and the participation of multidisciplinary teams made up of radiologists, pathologists, and gastroenterologists.

b. Patients with Barrett's oesophagus should follow the guidelines for surveillance intervals, which include getting regular endoscopic exams and histological analyses to track the disease's course and direct treatment decisions.

c. In order to guarantee accurate and repeatable diagnostic results, healthcare facilities performing Barrett's Oesophagus diagnostic evaluations should follow established protocols that include the use of quality assurance measures, strict biopsy acquisition techniques, and competent histopathological processing.

By successfully completing the diagnostic roadmap for Barrett's Oesophagus, non-invasive screening methods, endoscopic assessments, and histopathological analyses are all integrated and can be used to accurately identify and characterise the condition, which in turn informs management plans and surveillance procedures.

For Barrett's Oesophagus, additional diagnostic insights and solutions to diagnostic conundrums may be provided by advanced imaging modalities like confocal laser endomicroscopy or narrow-band imaging. This will enhance the diagnostic toolkit in the event of inconclusive diagnostic findings or inconsistent results between non-invasive screening tests and endoscopic evaluations.

Following our exploration of the complex terrain of Barrett's Oesophagus diagnostic procedures and tests, the next chapter will address treatment options and management techniques, clarifying the critical function that a precise diagnosis plays in maximising clinical results and promoting patient-centered care.

The Barrett's Oesophagus Mastery Bible: The fourth chapter of your blueprint, "Therapeutic Modalities and Management Strategies," deals with Barrett's oesophagus management in detail.

Prevalence and Statistics

Barrett's oesophagus (BE) is a premalignant disorder in which the distal oesophagus develops metaplastic columnar epithelium in place of normal squamous epithelium. This illness greatly raises the chance of developing esophageal cancer and is closely linked to gastroesophageal reflux disease (GERD) (EAC). For management and prevention initiatives to be effective, it is essential to comprehend the prevalence of BE and its effects on various demographic groups.

Over the past few decades, Barrett's oesophagus has become more common and has varied effects on different demographic groups.

Research has continuously indicated an increase in BE prevalence, with a discernible rise in Western nations. The prevalence of BE grew from 3.3 percent in 1996 to 6.8 percent in 2005 in the United States, according to a study by Hvid-Jensen et al. (2011). This alarming nearly twofold increase in incidence in a short amount of time emphasises the necessity for all-encompassing management approaches.

Numerous variables have been linked to the growth in BE prevalence, including the rising incidence of obesity and the GERD that goes along with it, which is a major risk factor for BE. The high fat and low fibre content of the Western diet has also been linked to the development of BE, which adds to the disease's prevalence.

Furthermore, research has shown that differences in BE prevalence according to gender and ethnicity exist. Studies have repeatedly shown that men are more likely than women to have BE, with some indicating that the frequency in men may be two or even three times higher. More research is necessary to determine the causes of this gender gap, which could be related to behavioural, genetic, or hormonal variables.

There have also been noted ethnic differences in BE prevalence, with Caucasian people showing a higher incidence than other ethnic groupings. This discrepancy could be attributed to environmental circumstances, genetic predisposition, or both.

Although there is no denying that BE is more common now, some experts are concerned about overdiagnosis and the possible effects of surveillance bias. The identification of non-progressive or clinically unimportant instances of BE is referred to as overdiagnosis, which results in needless treatments and higher healthcare expenses. Conversely, surveillance bias may arise from heightened awareness and screening, resulting in the identification of asymptomatic patients that might not proceed to more advanced stages.

Although these worries are legitimate, overdiagnosis and monitoring bias are not the only reasons for the significant increase in BE prevalence. A strong case can be made for the true rise in BE cases given the rise in obesity rates, dietary modifications, and the changing epidemiology of GERD. Accurate prevalence data are crucial because of the high correlation that exists between BE and EAC, which calls for the proactive identification and therapy of BE patients.

Longitudinal population-based studies have shown an increase in the incidence of EAC, a well-documented result of untreated or improperly managed BE, lending further credence to the assertion that BE prevalence is rising. The increase in BE prevalence that has been seen is consistent with the rise in EAC cases, which emphasises how urgent it is to address this public health issue.

In conclusion, there is evidence that the prevalence of Barrett's oesophagus has increased, especially in Western nations, and that there are differences according to gender and ethnicity. The significant increase in BE prevalence is a result of shifting GERD, obesity, and eating patterns, notwithstanding legitimate worries about overdiagnosis and surveillance bias. In order to effectively manage and implement preventative initiatives to reduce the risk of esophageal adenocarcinoma, it is necessary to address this shift. Accurate prevalence data play a vital role in informing public health interventions and providing tailored patient treatment.

The following chapters will delve deeper into the complex terrain of Barrett's oesophagus and examine the novel techniques and comprehensive care strategies targeted at improving outcomes for patients with this ailment.

Barrett's Esophagus Mastery Bible: The Ultimate Guide to Chapter 3 of Barrett's Esophagus Management, "Risk Stratification and Surveillance Protocols," is the next chapter.

Complications and Associated Conditions

Creating a thorough management plan for Barrett's oesophagus (BE) requires a thorough understanding of the possible side effects and comorbidities. This section will clarify the complex network of health implications that BE patients may experience, illuminating the complex character of this premalignant illness.

The inventory that follows provides a thorough summary of the various health consequences connected to BE by outlining potential problems and related conditions:

a. Becoming esophageal adenocarcinoma is the most serious and feared side effect of BE. EAC may arise as a result of the metaplastic epithelium changing into dysplastic and then cancerous cells. BE patients have a much higher risk of EAC than the general population, which highlights the urgent need for close observation and prompt care. The transition from BE to EAC emphasises how urgently comprehensive management plans must be implemented in order to stop cancer's potentially lethal end.

b. The cellular alterations and persistent inflammation linked to BE may cause esophageal strictures to form. The buildup of fibrous tissue in the lining of the oesophagus causes these strictures, which constrict the lumen of the oesophagus. Dysphagia, odynophagia, and a higher risk of food impaction are symptoms of restriction development that can seriously impair a person's quality of life. Endoscopic dilation or, in extreme situations, surgical intervention to relieve the esophageal narrowing may be necessary for the management of strictures.

c. BE is distinguished by the possibility of dysplastic alterations in the oesophagus epithelium, which can occur before the onset of EAC and range from low-grade dysplasia to high-grade dysplasia. Therapeutic therapies and risk assessment are greatly aided by the

31

detection and tracking of dysplastic alterations. Dysplasia patients have an increased risk of developing cancer, which emphasises the necessity of careful observation and individualised treatment plans to lessen this serious consequence.

d. Clinical literature has shown a correlation between BE and respiratory issues, specifically aspiration pneumonia and persistent cough. BE patients may have reflux of stomach contents into the respiratory system, which might result in pulmonary symptoms. The impact of respiratory difficulties on a person's health might increase the burden of BE and call for a multidisciplinary approach to comprehensive care.

e. Given that the pathophysiology and evolution of BE are influenced by the persistent reflux of stomach contents into the oesophagus, attention must be paid to the complex interaction between GERD and BE. The interdependence of both illnesses in clinical practise is shown by the critical role that effective GERD therapy plays in reducing the likelihood of complications related to BE.

f. Anemia and nutritional deficits may arise as a result of the long-term inflammation and possible bleeding linked to BE. Although less frequent in BE than in other esophageal disorders, gastrointestinal bleeding is nevertheless a cause for concern, requiring close observation and timely treatment of anaemia and nutritional abnormalities in those who are affected.

g. It's important to recognise the psychological toll that having a premalignant illness like BE can take. For those with BE, the constant threat of cancer, the requirement for routine monitoring, and the possibility of changing their way of life can all be extremely upsetting. Giving patients comprehensive treatment and support as they navigate the difficulties of BE requires an understanding of and attention to the psychological impact of the condition.

h. Extraesophageal symptoms, such as laryngopharyngeal reflux, a persistent cough, and tooth erosions, have been linked to BE. The range of health consequences associated with BE is expanded by these extraesophageal symptoms, highlighting the necessity of a thorough evaluation of related disorders in order to maximise patient management.

Prolonged cohort studies, meta-analyses, and clinical observations are just a few of the numerous clinical evidences that bolster the complex web of comorbidities and related illnesses associated with BE. The diverse range of health issues linked to BE is further highlighted by testimonies from people who have the disorder and medical professionals who assist in their care.

Clinical practise is directly impacted by a thorough awareness of the possible side effects and coexisting conditions of BE, which informs risk assessment, monitoring procedures, and customised treatment plans. The incorporation of this knowledge into patient care can enable medical providers to offer persons navigating the intricacies of BE individualised, comprehensive support.

The complex network of possible side effects and other illnesses that accompany BE highlights how diverse this premalignant illness is. In the next several chapters, we'll move our attention to outlining creative ways to improve outcomes for people with BE as well as evidence-based management practises.

Medical Management of Barrett's Oesophagus

Medications Explained

Understanding the drugs that are the foundation of Barrett's Oesophagus treatment is essential as we delve into the complex world of this condition's care. We can have a better understanding of these crucial drugs' mechanisms of action, possible adverse effects, and overall influence on Barrett's oesophagus management by being familiar with them.

Comprehending the primary drugs utilised in the management of Barrett's oesophagus is essential for individuals receiving care, medical professionals treating them, and patients. This knowledge is essential for efficient management since it enables people to choose their treatments with knowledge. Thus, a thorough investigation of these drugs is necessary to guarantee a solid understanding of their function in the treatment of Barrett's oesophagus.

List the Terms

To facilitate a clear and organized understanding of the medications involved, we will delineate and elucidate the following key terms:

1. Proton Pump Inhibitors (PPIs)
2. H2 Receptor Antagonists
3. Nonsteroidal Anti-Inflammatory Drugs (NSAIDs)
4. Antacids
5. Prokinetics
6. Cytoprotective Agents
7. Endoscopic Therapy

1. Proton Pump Inhibitors (PPIs)

A class of drugs known as proton pump inhibitors (PPIs) works by stopping the stomach's proton pump, which lowers the amount of acid produced. By doing this, proton pump inhibitors (PPIs) successfully reduce the symptoms of gastroesophageal reflux disease (GERD) and are essential in controlling and delaying the advancement of Barrett's oesophagus. Omeprazole, lansoprazole, esomeprazole, pantoprazole, and rabeprazole are a few examples of PPIs that are frequently prescribed.

Link to Real-world or Familiar Concepts

To understand the importance of PPIs in Barrett's Oesophagus management, consider how they work like a tap to regulate water flow. Similar to how shutting off the water supply decreases its flow, PPIs work by blocking the proton pump, which lowers stomach acid production and lessens the risk of acid reflux into the oesophagus. This practical comparison helps to clarify the workings of PPIs and their essential role in Barrett's oesophagus management.

2. H2 Receptor Antagonists

Another class of drugs called H2 receptor antagonists, or H2 blockers, reduces the production of stomach acid by selectively blocking the H2 receptors in the stomach. H2 receptor antagonists are useful in treating milder cases of acid reflux and can be used as supplementary therapy in conjunction with PPIs, despite their lower potency compared to PPIs.

Link to Real-world or Familiar Concepts

H2 receptor antagonists control the activity of the H2 receptors, which is similar to a dimmer switch controlling light intensity. This allows them to modify the generation of stomach acid. This comparison offers a meaningful example to understand how H2 receptor antagonists control acid reflux and how Barrett's oesophagus is affected by it.

3. Nonsteroidal Anti-Inflammatory Drugs (NSAIDs)

A class of pharmaceuticals called nonsteroidal anti-inflammatory drugs (NSAIDs) is frequently prescribed to treat pain and inflammation. Although their main purpose is not to treat Barrett's oesophagus per se, their capacity to harm the oesophageal mucosa emphasises the importance of using them carefully and sparingly in patients who have this illness.

Link to Real-world or Familiar Concepts

The way that NSAIDs affect the mucosa of the oesophagus is comparable to how abrasive materials affect sensitive surfaces. NSAIDs have the ability to irritate and harm the lining of the oesophagus, much like sandpaper can abrasion smooth surfaces. This highlights the significance of taking into account their impact on Barrett's Oesophagus therapy.

4. Antacids

Acid reflux symptoms can be quickly relieved by using over-the-counter antacids, which neutralise stomach acid. Antacids are useful for providing temporary relief and can be used as supplemental therapy in the management of milder cases of acid reflux, even though they are not as effective as PPIs or H2 receptor antagonists in reducing the generation of acid.

Link to Real-world or Familiar Concepts

Antacids work similarly to baking soda added to vinegar to create a neutral pH in that they neutralise acidic solutions by adding alkaline materials. This example helps to clarify how antacids relieve acid reflux symptoms in a concrete way, which facilitates understanding of their function in Barrett's oesophagus management.

5. Prokinetics

Prokinetic drugs increase the gastrointestinal tract's motility, which makes it easier for food to pass through the digestive system. Prokinetics can help people with reduced oesophageal motility clear refluxed material from their oesophagus and lower their risk of problems, even though their main function is not to manage Barrett's oesophagus.

Link to Real-world or Familiar Concepts

Prokinetics works like a conveyor belt that moves products along a production line quickly and efficiently while avoiding bottlenecks. Prokinetics, on the other hand, aid in the easy passage of food through the digestive system, avoiding stagnation and lessening the possibility of reflux and its aftereffects in those with Barrett's oesophagus.

6. Cytoprotective Agents

Drugs known as "cytoprotective drugs" shield the gastrointestinal tract's mucosal lining from harm while accelerating the healing process. Although cytoprotective drugs are not specifically designed to treat Barrett's oesophagus, they can be helpful in reducing the risk of oesophageal lining damage brought on by acid reflux and other irritants.

Link to Real-world or Familiar Concepts

Comparable to a varnish layer that protects wood from moisture and wear, the function of cytoprotective agents is akin to a barrier that keeps fragile surfaces safe. This comparison clarifies how cytoprotective drugs protect the mucosa lining the oesophagus and may be useful in treating Barrett's oesophagus.

7. Endoscopic Therapy

Endoscopic therapy is a group of minimally invasive techniques used to treat Barrett's oesophagus and its related problems. These operations are carried out via an endoscope. These operations could use methods like radiofrequency ablation (RFA) and endoscopic mucosal resection (EMR), which are meant to remove aberrant tissue and lower the chance that it will proceed to oesophageal cancer.

Link to Real-world or Familiar Concepts

Endoscopic therapy can be compared to fine instruments used in fine craftsmanship, such as a chisel used by a sculptor to carefully carve and shape minute features. This comparison illustrates the delicacy and accuracy of endoscopic treatments and clarifies their function in controlling Barrett's oesophagus and averting unfavourable consequences.

Conclusion

In conclusion, it is critical for everyone involved in the care of Barrett's oesophagus to have a solid grasp of the drugs utilised in its therapy. Through the explanation of each medication's mode of action, possible adverse effects, and practical equivalents, we hope to offer a thorough understanding of its function in the overall care of Barrett's oesophagus. With this information, patients, caregivers, and medical professionals can manage this difficult condition more effectively and make educated decisions.

Endoscopic Treatments

We must now move on to the topic of endoscopic therapies as we continue our thorough investigation of Barrett's oesophagus management. In order to address the underlying mucosal alterations and lower the risk of development to oesophageal cancer, endoscopic procedures are essential in the management of Barrett's oesophagus. Patients, caregivers, and healthcare professionals must all be aware of the subtleties of these endoscopic therapies in order for them to be able to make educated decisions and take an active role in the management of this complicated ailment.

The following list encapsulates the key endoscopic treatments for Barrett's Oesophagus:

1. Endoscopic Surveillance
2. Endoscopic Mucosal Resection (EMR)
3. Radiofrequency Ablation (RFA)
4. Cryotherapy
5. Photodynamic Therapy (PDT)
6. Endoscopic Submucosal Dissection (ESD)

a. A vital component of Barrett's oesophagus care is endoscopic monitoring, which tracks the disease's development, recognises dysplastic alterations, and directs further treatments. It entails routine endoscopic exams of the oesophagus, during which samples are taken from the impacted mucosa to determine whether dysplasia or cancer is present. This surveillance approach lowers the chance of advanced disease by enabling prompt action and early detection of high-risk changes.

b. EMR, or endoscopic mucosal resection, is a minimally invasive procedure used to remove aberrant portions of the oesophageal mucosa. The targeted tissue is removed either piecemeal or en bloc using specialised endoscopic devices, which enables the excision of dysplastic or early malignant tumours that are limited to the mucosal layer. EMR is a useful technique for Barrett's Oesophagus therapy since it can efficiently remove precancerous lesions and lower the chance that the illness will worsen.

c. An innovative technique in the endoscopic therapeutic arsenal for Barrett's oesophagus is radiofrequency ablation, or RFA. Using this method, the dysplastic cells are specifically destroyed by applying regulated heat energy to the aberrant oesophageal mucosa. Not only does RFA remove the current Barrett's epithelium, but it also encourages the normal, healthy oesophageal tissue to regrow. RFA is now considered the standard of care for the treatment of Barrett's oesophagus due to its effectiveness in slowing the progression of the disease and lowering the risk of oesophageal cancer.

d. Using the idea of extreme cold, cryotherapy, commonly referred to as cryoablation, ablates dysplastic or malignant tissue located within the oesophagus. Through the use of an endoscopic catheter, cryogenic agents—such as liquid nitrogen or carbon dioxide—are delivered to the targeted tissue, which is quickly frozen and then thawed, causing cellular damage and necrosis. Barrett's oesophagus can be effectively treated with cryotherapy in a variety of situations when typical endoscopic procedures may be difficult or unfeasible.

e. Cryotherapy, sometimes referred to as cryoablation, uses extremely low temperatures to destroy malignant or dysplastic tissue in the oesophagus. Through the use of an endoscopic catheter to administer cryogenic agents—such as carbon dioxide or liquid nitrogen—the targeted tissue is quickly frozen and then thawed, causing cellular damage and necrosis. When typical endoscopic procedures are difficult or impossible to use, cryotherapy provides a flexible and efficient treatment option for Barrett's oesophagus.

f. An sophisticated endoscopic procedure called endoscopic submucosal dissection, or ESD, is intended to enable en bloc resection of bigger, superficial gastrointestinal neoplasms, including those that originate within Barrett's oesophagus. In contrast to standard EMR,

ESD allows for accurate histological assessment and full excision by precisely dissecting lesions of any size or shape. Although technically complex, endoscopic subtraction has been shown to be promising in the treatment of early neoplastic lesions in Barrett's oesophagus, with the possibility of curative resection and decreased recurrence rates.

Numerous clinical studies and real-world experiences support the effectiveness of various endoscopic therapies in the management of Barrett's oesophagus. Several studies have shown that endoscopic treatments, especially RFA and EMR, can eliminate dysplastic alterations, lower the likelihood of the illness progressing, and enhance long-term outcomes for individuals with Barrett's oesophagus. Moreover, testimonies from patients who have had these operations highlight the important role endoscopic therapies play in reducing the severity of this illness and providing hope for a good prognosis.

These endoscopic procedures have real-world uses outside of clinical practise that lead to observable improvements in patient outcomes. Healthcare professionals can optimise the time and selection of therapeutic interventions by proactively identifying and addressing disease progression by incorporating endoscopic surveillance into the long-term management of Barrett's Oesophagus. With customised methods to the removal of dysplastic and neoplastic alterations in the oesophagus, EMR, RFA, PDT, and ESD provide patients with the chance for enhanced survival and curative treatment. When used carefully, these endoscopic procedures significantly lessen the symptoms of Barrett's oesophagus and lower the risk of oesophageal cancer.

When we move from explaining specific endoscopic procedures to discussing how they all affect the overall care of Barrett's oesophagus, it becomes critical to understand how these interventions interact with the larger care chain. Endoscopic monitoring, EMR, RFA, cryotherapy, PDT, and ESD are all seamlessly integrated to support a multimodal approach to Barrett's oesophagus management that puts an emphasis on early detection, accurate intervention, and long-term disease control. This well-coordinated approach perfectly captures the holistic management philosophy that is necessary to maximise patient outcomes and lessen the aftereffects of this difficult condition.

In summary, the range of endoscopic procedures available for treating Barrett's oesophagus is indicative of the rapidly evolving fields of precision medicine and therapeutic innovation. When endoscopic surveillance is combined with a variety of cutting-edge therapies, patients and healthcare professionals have a powerful toolkit to fight Barrett's oesophagus. In the fields of gastroenterology and cancer, the prudent use of endoscopic treatments not only heralds a new era of individualised, patient-centered care but also presents potential for disease eradication and progression mitigation.

Surgical Options

After navigating the complexities of endoscopic treatments for Barrett's oesophagus, a thorough investigation of the surgical options to be taken into consideration for the treatment of this complicated ailment is necessary. When it comes to severe disease, high-grade dysplasia, or situations that are resistant to treatment, surgical interventions are essential, even if endoscopic therapies are the foundation of first therapeutic techniques. The list that follows provides a thorough summary of the surgical techniques related to Barrett's oesophagus care, together with information on their indications, specifics of the procedure, and results in the clinic.

The surgical methods available for treating Barrett's oesophagus comprise a range of techniques customised to meet the unique requirements and disease features of each patient. Among the principal surgical modalities are:

1. Endoscopic Resection and Surgical Resection
2. Oesophagectomy
3. Anti-reflux Surgery

a. There are two main surgical procedures for Barrett's oesophagus: endoscopic resection and surgical resection. Both have advantages and disadvantages that should be taken into account while managing advanced disease. Endoscopic resection methods, such endoscopic submucosal dissection (ESD) and endoscopic mucosal resection (EMR), are generally used as a less intrusive substitute for standard surgical resection in the excision of early neoplastic lesions that are limited to the mucosal layer. On the other hand, in cases of deeper involvement of the mucosa, a greater disease load, or the development of invasive carcinoma, surgical resection—typically performed as a partial oesophagectomy or segmental resection—becomes essential. The choice between endoscopic and surgical resection is based on a thorough evaluation of the patient's comorbidities, the extent of the disease, and the likelihood of receiving a curative treatment.

b. The gold standard surgical treatment for Barrett's Oesophagus involving invasive adenocarcinoma, intramucosal carcinoma, or high-grade dysplasia is oesophagectomy. In order to address possible metastatic spread, this comprehensive treatment frequently includes the removal of a portion of the oesophagus along with a lymphadenectomy. There are several ways to execute an oesophagectomy, such as open surgery, robotic-assisted procedures, and minimally invasive techniques. Each of these methods has advantages over the other in terms of long-term results, surgical precision, and postoperative recovery. With the ultimate goal of attaining total eradication of neoplastic alterations while maintaining functional integrity, the best oesophagectomy strategy is determined based on patient-specific criteria, disease features, and institutional expertise.

c. When Barrett's Oesophagus is present, the co-existence of gastroesophageal reflux disease (GERD) frequently calls for a collaborative strategy to managing the condition, which may include anti-reflux surgery. The cornerstone of anti-reflux surgical therapies, fundoplication (including both laparoscopic Nissen and partial fundoplication) aims to reinforce the lower oesophageal sphincter and restore the physiological barrier against reflux. Anti-reflux surgery reduces the risk factors for Barrett's esophagitis formation and progression in addition to relieving symptoms by treating the underlying reflux pathology. The careful incorporation of anti-reflux surgery into the all-encompassing Barrett's Oesophagus management paradigm highlights the procedure's importance in reducing the risk of recurrence and maximising long-term results.

A substantial amount of clinical evidence and patient testimonials support the effectiveness of surgical options in the management of Barrett's oesophagus. These resources also reinforce the critical role that surgical interventions play in managing advanced disease and reducing the risk of oesophageal adenocarcinoma. Prospective trials and long-term research have shown that oesophagectomy can be a curative treatment for early invasive cancer and high-grade dysplasia, leading to better survival rates and longer intervals without disease. Testimonials from patients who have had anti-reflux surgery or surgical resection emphasise the profoundly positive effects these procedures have had on their quality of life and demonstrate how comprehensive surgical management is in treating both the functional and oncological aspects of Barrett's oesophagus.

Surgical alternatives have practical uses not only in disease eradication but also in patient-centered treatment and holistic illness management. When used carefully, endoscopic and surgical resection can be curative and provide long-term disease control, especially when early neoplastic lesions and confined illness are present. As the ultimate surgical procedure, oesophagectomy requires a multidisciplinary strategy that includes oncological surveillance, perioperative care, and surgical competence in order to maximise patient outcomes and reduce the risk of disease recurrence. By treating the underlying reflux pathology and reducing the risk of disease development, anti-reflux surgery, when combined with endoscopic and surgical procedures, strengthens the continuity of care for Barrett's oesophagus and emphasises the comprehensive character of surgical management.

Surgical alternatives and their combined effects on the overall therapy of Barrett's oesophagus are becoming more and more important, and it is critical to understand how endoscopic, surgical, and medicinal modalities work together to maximise patient outcomes. Curative therapy, functional restoration, and long-term disease control are given priority in the multifaceted management of Barrett's oesophagus, which is made possible by the smooth integration of endoscopic resection, surgical resection, oesophagectomy, and anti-reflux surgery. Personalized, patient-centered care is crucial for managing Barrett's oesophagus, and this well-coordinated approach highlights how important it is to take a multidisciplinary, holistic approach to disease management.

To sum up, the range of surgical treatments available for Barrett's Oesophagus represents the advancement of precision medicine and therapeutic innovation, providing a customised approach to treating high-grade dysplasia, advanced illness, and refractory cases. Through the integration of endoscopic, surgical, and anti-reflux therapies, patients and healthcare providers are better prepared to tackle the obstacles presented by Barrett's Oesophagus, leading to the dawn of a new era in individualised, multidisciplinary gastroenterology and cancer care.

Follow-up Care and Monitoring

Our main objective in this part is to clarify the vital significance of routine follow-up care and monitoring in the all-encompassing management of Barrett's oesophagus. Readers will have a clear knowledge of the benefits of follow-up care, what makes for efficient monitoring, and how important longitudinal surveillance is to slowing the progression of the disease and improving patient outcomes at the end of this chapter.

Prior to discussing the details of follow-up treatment and monitoring, it is critical to emphasise the essential requirements for effective patient management. The natural history of Barrett's oesophagus should be thoroughly understood, neoplastic progression risk stratification should be familiarised with, and endoscopic, surgical, and pharmacological therapies should be seamlessly integrated into the continuum of therapy. Furthermore, the formation of a multidisciplinary team consisting of surgeons, gastroenterologists, pathologists, and oncologists is essential to the comprehensive care of patients suffering with Barrett's oesophagus.

A systematic approach to the monitoring and follow-up care of patients with Barrett's oesophagus involves a step-by-step plan that starts with the post-interventional surveillance after endoscopic or surgical procedures. The monitoring of the disease's evolution over time, early detection of neoplastic transformation, and prudent use of therapeutic measures to reduce the risk of oesophageal adenocarcinoma are the next steps. In order to maximise patient outcomes and reduce the burden of advanced disease, the main goals are to accomplish early detection, prompt management, and sustained disease control.

1. The foundation of follow-up care is the start of post-procedural observation once endoscopic or surgical procedures are finished. This stage includes a thorough evaluation of the procedure's results, a

determination of any possible consequences, and the creation of a customised follow-up plan to track the progression of the disease and identify any lingering or recurrent neoplastic abnormalities. Endoscopic surveillance allows for the resolution of dysplastic alterations, the identification of metachronous lesions, and a thorough assessment of mucosal healing. It includes high-definition white-light endoscopy as well as complementary imaging modalities like chromoendoscopy and narrow-band imaging. Simultaneously, an early detection of post-procedural problems, including bleeding, perforation, or stricture formation, calls for aggressive therapy in order to guarantee both the best possible outcome for the patient and the success of the procedure.

2. Barrett's Oesophagus longitudinal surveillance encompasses a lifetime commitment to disease monitoring and risk assessment, going beyond the immediate post-procedural phase. This includes the use of sophisticated imaging technologies, such as volumetric laser endomicroscopy and confocal laser endomicroscopy, to improve the detection of neoplastic changes at a submucosal level, as well as routine endoscopic evaluations at predetermined intervals and the histopathological assessment of mucosal biopsies. The prudent utilisation of risk stratification instruments, like the Barrett's Oesophagus Surveillance Pathway, facilitates customization of surveillance intervals according to the risk profile of each patient. This approach maximises the distribution of healthcare resources and reduces the load of overly intrusive surveillance in low-risk groups.

3. Proactively identifying neoplastic development and promptly implementing adaptive treatment strategies are essential for the comprehensive care of Barrett's oesophagus. This includes the endoscopic removal of early neoplastic lesions or dysplastic foci by means of methods including cryotherapy, radiofrequency ablation, and endoscopic mucosal resection, which reduces the likelihood of the illness progressing and invasive carcinoma developing. Moreover, a

comprehensive approach to disease treatment is ensured by the smooth integration of surgical resection, oesophagectomy, or anti-reflux surgery within the monitoring paradigm, addressing the growing disease burden or the return of dysplastic alterations.

- Tip 1: Stress the critical role that patient education and participation play in encouraging patients to follow the recommended surveillance intervals and make lifestyle changes, which in turn promotes a cooperative relationship between patients and healthcare professionals.

- Tip 2: Promote the incorporation of digital health technology, such as platforms for remote patient monitoring and telemonitoring, to improve patient compliance and make follow-up care more accessible, especially for underprivileged or rural populations.

- Warning 1: Warn against becoming complacent with regard to monitoring procedures, emphasising the need for thorough endoscopic examinations and histological analyses in order to guarantee the thorough identification of neoplastic alterations and the prompt administration of therapeutic measures.

The successful execution of post-interventional surveillance and longitudinal monitoring is confirmed by means of the thorough recording of endoscopic observations, histological evaluations, and the development of adaptable treatment plans. Furthermore, the positive patient outcomes—such as the persistent regression of dysplastic changes, the early identification of neoplastic progression, and the appropriate distribution of therapeutic interventions to maximise disease control and patient survival—underline the validity of effective follow-up care and monitoring.

When surgical results are not as good as expected or tumour changes are discovered while monitoring a patient, a multidisciplinary tumour board composed of surgeons, oncologists, and gastroenterologists should be formed in order to discuss potential adaptive treatment plans and to facilitate a smooth transition to the next stage of the patient's care. Furthermore, the prudent utilisation of sophisticated endoscopic methods, such as optical coherence tomography and endoscopic ultrasound, facilitates the creation of customised therapy algorithms to handle intricate neoplastic situations and the thorough evaluation of the degree of disease.

To sum up, the adoption of a thorough monitoring and follow-up care model for patients with Barrett's oesophagus exemplifies the integration of precision medicine and patient-centered care, promoting early identification, prompt intervention, and long-term disease management. Through adherence to the recommended surveillance intervals, the utilisation of advanced imaging technologies, and the integration of adaptive therapeutic interventions, patients and healthcare providers can effectively manage the intricacies of Barrett's Oesophagus and usher in a new era of personalised, multidisciplinary gastroenterology and oncology care.

Addressing Complications

Oesophageal adenocarcinoma risk is higher in patients with Barrett's Oesophagus, a disorder marked by the metaplastic columnar epithelium of the lower oesophagus replacing the typical squamous epithelium of the oesophagus. Although surveillance and early intervention for neoplastic advancement are frequently the main focus of care strategies, it is crucial to recognise and address any potential complications that may arise during Barrett's Oesophagus management. The significance of proactive treatment measures in reducing the development and impact of these complications cannot be overstated, as they can have a substantial influence on patient outcomes and quality of life if left mismanaged.

The main problem at hand is the complex nature of difficulties related to the therapy of Barrett's oesophagus. These problems cover a wide range of issues, from adverse effects that occur during therapeutic procedures to the complex interactions between dysplastic alterations, chronic reflux, and oesophageal cancer development. Moreover, a thorough grasp of these consequences and a proactive approach to their management are required due to the possible effects they may have on patient morbidity, mortality, and the use of healthcare resources.

Negative outcomes may occur if Barrett's oesophagus management-related complications are not well managed. Long hospital stays, repeated operations, and a reduced quality of life are possible for patients. Furthermore, the development of complications—such as haemorrhage, strictures, or malignant transformation—can have a substantial effect on long-term survival and add to the growing cost of healthcare that comes with advanced disease states. Furthermore, it is impossible to overstate the psychological and emotional toll that the uncertainty and difficulty of addressing these issues takes on patients and their families.

A multifaceted strategy is necessary to effectively alleviate the problems that have been discovered. This means taking proactive steps to stop complications from developing, recognising and treating issues early on, and putting in place specialised treatment plans to deal with the unique characteristics of each problem. In addition, a patient-centered strategy that includes both shared decision-making and thorough patient education is essential for encouraging cooperation between patients and healthcare professionals as they navigate the challenges of managing these issues.

Strategies for managing complications must be implemented seamlessly within the current Barrett's Oesophagus care paradigm. This includes creating standardised protocols for the early detection and management of complications, forming multidisciplinary care teams to guarantee a comprehensive and coordinated approach to managing complications, and incorporating extensive risk stratification tools to identify patients at heightened risk of developing complications.

Clinical experience and available data both support the effectiveness of proactive therapy in reducing the risk of problems related to Barrett's oesophagus. Research has indicated that the adoption of standardised monitoring procedures, timely identification and management of procedural adverse events, and the incorporation of patient support initiatives have resulted in decreased rates of complications, enhanced patient contentment, and optimal use of available resources. Additionally, with the proactive management of these issues, predictive modelling based on these outcomes predicts a significant decrease in the burden of complications and a corresponding improvement in patient outcomes.

Although the suggested method outlines a thorough plan to handle issues related to Barrett's oesophagus care, other options should be taken into account. These could involve investigating new therapeutic approaches to reduce the chance of complications, incorporating digital health technologies for early detection of complications and remote patient monitoring, and carefully assessing pharmacological and lifestyle interventions to stop complications in high-risk groups.

Understanding the complex relationship between the underlying ailment and any potential consequences is essential as we delve into the intricacies of managing Barrett's Oesophagus. We can maximise patient outcomes, reduce the burden of advanced disease states, and promote a patient-centered strategy that places a high priority on comprehensive care and ongoing disease control by proactively managing these complications. The details of each complication, customised management plans, and the critical role that teamwork in healthcare delivery plays in negotiating the complexities of Barrett's oesophagus care will all be thoroughly covered in the chapters to follow.

Interpreting Medical Jargon

It's critical for people with Barrett's oesophagus diagnoses to comprehend medical jargon. A lay reader may find it difficult to understand the abundance of medical jargon and concepts used due to the condition's intricacy and how it is managed. This chapter seeks to give patients and their caregivers the knowledge they need to properly engage with the content of this book by demystifying these terms and offering concise explanations connected to everyday concepts.

In order to promote a thorough comprehension of Barrett's Oesophagus and its treatment, the following terminology will be clarified and thoroughly examined:

1. Barrett's Oesophagus
2. Metaplasia
3. Neoplastic progression
4. Dysplastic changes
5. Oesophageal adenocarcinoma
6. Adverse events
7. Reflux
8. Strictures
9. Bleeding
10. Multidisciplinary care teams

1. Barrett's Oesophagus is a condition marked by the metaplastic columnar epithelium of the lower oesophagus replacing the normal squamous epithelium. This alteration is a major risk factor for the development of oesophageal adenocarcinoma and is frequently linked to chronic gastroesophageal reflux disease (GERD).

2. The reversible transformation known as "metaplasia" occurs when one adult cell type is replaced by another. When referring to Barrett's Oesophagus, the term "metaplasia" refers to the change from the typical lower oesophageal squamous epithelium into metaplastic columnar epithelium.

3. When discussing Barrett's oesophagus, the term "neoplastic progression" refers to the evolution of malignant cellular alterations within the metaplastic epithelium that eventually result in the creation of oesophageal adenocarcinoma.

4. Dysplastic alterations indicate aberrant, precancerous cellular alterations in the oesophageal metaplastic epithelium. These modifications point to a higher chance that the condition may proceed to oesophageal cancer.

5. A malignant tumour called oesophageal adenocarcinoma develops in the glandular tissue of the lower oesophagus. It is a serious side effect of Barrett's oesophagus that, if not identified and treated quickly, is linked to a bad prognosis.

6. Unwanted or unfavourable outcomes that follow therapeutic therapies or procedures are referred to as adverse events. Adverse occurrences in the context of managing Barrett's oesophagus may include surgical or endoscopic procedure-related problems.

7. Reflux, especially gastroesophageal reflux, is the backflow of stomach contents into the oesophagus. It frequently causes symptoms including regurgitation, heartburn, and pain in the chest. It frequently occurs before Barrett's oesophagus develops.

8. Strictures are constricted sections of the oesophagus that are frequently brought on by long-term inflammation and scarring. Strictures in the setting of Barrett's Oesophagus can make swallowing difficult and necessitate medical procedures to relieve symptoms.

9. A number of conditions, such as ulcers, inflammation, or cancerous tumours, can cause bleeding inside the oesophagus. Bleeding in the context of Barrett's Oesophagus can appear as a complication of advanced disease and can have major health consequences for the patient.

10. A wide range of medical specialists, including radiologists, pathologists, gastroenterologists, surgeons, oncologists, and others, work together in multidisciplinary care teams to create and carry out

comprehensive treatment plans for patients with complicated medical conditions like Barrett's oesophagus.

Making connections between these unfamiliar medical jargon and well-known ideas can help with understanding. One way to conceptualise and comprehend metaplasia is to compare it to the process of converting a building to serve a different purpose. Similarly, the oesophageal epithelium's transition to a distinct cell type signifies a shift in function, although one that occurs at the cellular level. Adverse events that occur after therapeutic interventions might be likened to unforeseen obstacles that arise throughout a voyage, emphasising the necessity for cautious navigation and management.

Patients and their caregivers can better comprehend the complexities of Barrett's oesophagus and its management by making connections between these terms and everyday ideas. This will enable them to take an active role in conversations with healthcare providers and make well-informed decisions about their care.

Navigating the Healthcare System

This chapter's main goal is to give people with Barrett's oesophagus a thorough overview of how to use the healthcare system so that their disease is managed as best they can. This chapter seeks to enable patients and their caregivers to take an active role in their care, make educated decisions, and obtain the support and resources they need by demystifying the intricacies of healthcare systems and procedures.

In order to begin managing Barrett's oesophagus, people will need to get access to relevant medical information, have a solid awareness of their illness, and adopt a proactive approach to advocating for their own health needs. To successfully navigate the healthcare system, one must also be conversant with medical language and be willing to speak effectively with medical specialists.

Understanding the roles of healthcare professionals, getting the right medical attention, coordinating different parts of treatment, and fighting for individualised care are all important components of navigating the healthcare system. Building a solid foundation of knowledge about Barrett's oesophagus is the first step in the process, which also includes speaking with medical professionals, getting access to diagnostic and treatment options, and, in the end, creating a customised management plan that takes the needs and preferences of the patient into account.

1. To navigate the healthcare system, one must have a thorough awareness of the environment in which healthcare is provided. The roles of various healthcare professionals, including gastroenterologists, surgeons, oncologists, and primary care physicians, should be understood by patients and caregivers. Gaining understanding of how diagnostic centres, treatment facilities, and support services operate can also help in successfully navigating the healthcare system.

2. Achieving smooth communication with healthcare providers requires organising and keeping an extensive record of medical history,

diagnostic findings, treatment plans, and prescription schedules. Patients should keep an orderly medical file with pertinent contact information, insurance information, and a history of all previous and current treatments.

3. Effective cooperation with healthcare providers requires the development of good communication skills to express symptoms, concerns, and treatment preferences. When faced with medical jargon or difficult topics, patients should actively participate in talks, ask important questions, and seek clarification. Developing a cooperative connection with medical professionals helps to promote a patient-centered care model.

4. Making educated decisions requires an understanding of the intent, methodology, and possible results of diagnostic procedures such endoscopies, biopsies, and imaging tests. Patients should actively participate in shared decision-making with their healthcare team and be fully educated about the risks, advantages, and alternatives of diagnostic tests.

5. Patients can take an active role in treatment planning by having access to information about different treatment modalities, such as endoscopic procedures, surgical choices, and surveillance regimens. Making educated decisions on the management of Barrett's oesophagus requires weighing the possible advantages, dangers, and long-term effects of various treatment modalities.

6. Communicating individual preferences, values, and goals to healthcare providers is a crucial part of advocating for individualised treatment. In order to receive personalised care that fits their lifestyle and general well-being, patients should actively participate in care planning, communicate their treatment preferences, and look for such approaches.

- Learn more about Barrett's oesophagus and become acquainted with reliable resources to improve your comprehension of the illness and how to treat it.

- Keep the lines of communication open with your healthcare providers to make sure any of your queries and worries are taken care of.

- When it comes to Barrett's oesophagus, stay away from sensationalised or false material that can be found online and instead rely on reliable, evidence-based sources that have the support of respectable medical associations.

- For individualised medical advice and management, seek the counsel of licenced healthcare professionals rather than self-diagnosing and treating yourself.

A collaborative relationship with healthcare providers, informed decision-making about treatment options, and the creation of a personalised management plan that is in line with individual needs and preferences can all serve as evidence of a successful navigation of the healthcare system for the management of Barrett's oesophagus. Furthermore, getting the right support services, knowing what insurance covers, and actively participating in shared decision-making across the care continuum are all necessary for successful navigation.

Patients and caregivers should consult patient advocacy organisations, social workers, or healthcare navigators for assistance if they experience difficulties navigating the healthcare system, including difficulty accessing specialised care, conflicting treatment recommendations, or barriers to communication with healthcare providers. These tools can offer helpful assistance in overcoming challenges and skillfully handling challenging healthcare situations.

In summary, navigating the healthcare system for the best management of Barrett's oesophagus requires a proactive, knowledgeable strategy that includes good communication, teamwork with medical specialists, and support for individualised treatment. Through the provision of information and skills to enable individuals to effectively navigate the healthcare system, this chapter seeks to enable patients and caregivers to take an active role in their care and to attain positive results in the management of Barrett's oesophagus.

Dietary Interventions and Nutrition

The Barrett's Diet: An Overview

Foods to Embrace

It is impossible to overestimate the importance of dietary decisions in the management of Barrett's oesophagus. Making the correct dietary choices can be extremely important for symptom relief, inflammation reduction, and esophageal health promotion. This chapter attempts to give a thorough list of foods that are good for people with Barrett's oesophagus as well as an exploration of the scientific basis for their benefits.

The following list encapsulates key foods that have shown promise in supporting the management of Barrett's esophagus:

1. Whole Grains
2. Leafy Greens
3. Lean Protein Sources
4. Fresh Fruits
5. Healthy Fats

Whole Grains

a. Whole grains are high in fibre, vitamins, and minerals. Examples of these are brown rice, quinoa, and whole wheat. Their high fibre content aids in digestion and helps shield against constipation, which is a typical problem for people suffering with Barrett's oesophagus. Furthermore, whole grains include antioxidants and phytochemicals that have anti-inflammatory qualities that can help lessen esophageal inflammation linked to Barrett's oesophagus.

b. Research indicates that eating a diet high in whole grains reduces the chance of getting gastroesophageal reflux disease (GERD), a disorder that is closely related to Barrett's oesophagus. Whole grains' high fibre content serves as a prebiotic, encouraging the development of good gut bacteria and supporting the maintenance of a balanced gut microbiome, which is essential for digestive health in general.

c. Patients with Barrett's oesophagus who have cut whole grains into their meals attest to a reduction in symptoms of acid reflux and heartburn. Moreover, people with a history of Barrett's oesophagus who routinely eat whole grains along with other healthy lifestyle changes have shown a decreased risk of the condition progressing.

d. Real-World Uses: Whole grain bread can be substituted for white bread, whole grain pasta can be chosen over refined pasta, and whole grain cereals or oats can be added to breakfast routines to help incorporate whole grains into a regular diet.

Leafy Greens

a. Vegetables that are rich in vitamins, minerals, and phytochemicals, such as spinach, kale, and collard greens, offer a host of health advantages. Their high fibre content helps prevent constipation and encourage regular bowel movements, which is especially advantageous for those who have Barrett's oesophagus.

b. Antioxidants found in leafy greens, such vitamin C and beta-carotene, have anti-inflammatory properties that may help lower esophageal inflammation and shield the oesophagus from oxidative stress, which is a major cause of esophageal damage in Barrett's oesophagus.

c. Research has demonstrated a link between eating more leafy greens and a lower incidence of esophageal adenocarcinoma, a serious Barrett's oesophagus problem. Furthermore, diets high in leafy greens are associated with a lower incidence of GERD symptoms, which may slow the advancement of Barrett's oesophagus, according to epidemiological research.

d. Practical Applications: There are many different ways to include leafy greens in meals. Some of them include adding them to salads, sautéing them as a side dish, blending them into smoothies, or adding them to soups and stews.

Lean Protein Sources

a. Fish, poultry, tofu, and legumes are examples of lean protein sources that are essential to a diet that is friendly to Barrett's oesophagus. Because these protein sources are low in fat, they are less likely to aggravate symptoms like heartburn and acid reflux, which are frequent in people with Barrett's oesophagus.

b. Lean protein consumption contributes vital amino acids required for muscle maintenance and tissue repair, promoting general health and facilitating the healing of Barrett's esophageal tissue.

c. Research has indicated that eating lean protein sources may help to alleviate GERD symptoms, which may help to control Barrett's oesophagus indirectly. A diet high in lean proteins can also help with weight control, since obesity and being overweight are recognised risk factors for the advancement of Barrett's oesophagus.

d. Practical Applications: Meals including lean protein sources can be prepared in a number of ways, including baking, steaming, and grilling. You can vary the sources of protein in your diet by replacing red meat with lean poultry or adding plant-based protein options like beans and tofu.

Fresh Fruits

a. For those with Barrett's oesophagus, fresh fruits like apples, bananas, and melons provide a multitude of health benefits. These fruits may help relieve Barrett's oesophagus symptoms and improve overall digestive health since they are high in fibre, vitamins, and antioxidants.

b. Fruits' high fibre content helps control bowel motions and increases satiety, which lowers the risk of overeating, which aggravates acid reflux and heartburn. In addition, fruits' natural sugars offer a healthier substitute for processed sweets, helping with glycemic control and weight management.

c. Regular consumption of fresh fruits is linked to a lower risk of esophageal adenocarcinoma, which is a persuasive consideration for people who already have Barrett's oesophagus, according to epidemiological research. Fruits' anti-inflammatory and antioxidant qualities can potentially help reduce oxidative stress and esophageal inflammation.

d. Practical Applications: Simple tactics like eating fresh fruits as snacks, including them into breakfast dishes, and putting them in fruit salads or smoothies can help include fresh fruits in the diet on a regular basis.

Healthy Fats

a. For those with Barrett's oesophagus, healthy fats like those in avocados, nuts, seeds, and olive oil are crucial parts of a balanced diet. In addition to offering a concentrated source of energy, these fats aid in the absorption of fat-soluble vitamins, which are vital for good health in general.

b. The anti-inflammatory properties of monounsaturated and polyunsaturated fats found in healthy fat sources may help to lessen esophageal inflammation and slow the development of Barrett's oesophagus.

c. Because good fats are less likely than their saturated counterparts to cause acid reflux and heartburn, research has shown that consuming them may help reduce the symptoms of GERD. Furthermore, including healthy fats in the diet can help with weight management and satiety, which addresses a major risk factor for Barrett's oesophagus.

d. Practical Applications: Nuts and seeds can be added to snacks and meals, avocados can be used as a versatile ingredient in dishes, and olive oil can be used for cooking and salad dressings. These are just a few ways to include healthy fats in the diet.

:

Including these health-promoting foods in the diet provides a comprehensive strategy for Barrett's oesophagus management. As we continue to explore the nuances of dietary management, it is clear that the combination of these dietary elements together with other lifestyle changes has potential to provide all-encompassing support for people coping with the complications of Barrett's oesophagus. We will continue to explore the many approaches to maximising esophageal health in the upcoming chapters, emphasising the critical role that dietary treatments play in this process.

Foods to Avoid

Knowing which foods can aggravate symptoms and cause esophageal inflammation is crucial for the comprehensive therapy of Barrett's oesophagus. In this chapter, a thorough list of foods to avoid is attempted to be outlined, together with information on any possible negative consequences and the underlying mechanisms that make certain meals inappropriate for people with Barrett's oesophagus.

Important items that have been demonstrated to worsen symptoms and increase esophageal inflammation in people with Barrett's oesophagus are summarised in the list below:

1. Spicy Foods
2. Citrus Fruits
3. Carbonated Beverages
4. High-fat Foods
5. Processed and Fried Foods

Spicy Foods

a. Foods that are considered spicy due to their high content of capsaicin and other volatile compounds have been linked to heartburn and acid reflux symptoms, which can worsen esophageal pain in people who have Barrett's oesophagus. Spicy food consumption may cause the lower esophageal sphincter (LES) to relax, which may allow stomach contents to reflux into the oesophagus and worsen esophageal inflammation.

b. Research has indicated that consuming spicy food is linked to more frequent acid reflux episodes, which may accelerate the development of Barrett's oesophagus and its related consequences. Moreover, spicy foods' irritating properties can directly cause esophageal pain and inflammation, therefore people who are managing Barrett's oesophagus should exercise caution when consuming them.

c. : Research from clinical studies and patient-reported outcomes has repeatedly shown how spicy meals exacerbate heartburn and acid reflux symptoms in people with Barrett's oesophagus. Patients who have reduced or stopped eating spicy meals attest to a decrease in esophageal discomfort as well as an improvement in the management of their symptoms.

d. Practical Applications: It is possible to prevent or minimise the aggravation of esophageal symptoms by avoiding or consuming spicy foods in moderation and by carefully planning meals and using softer substitutes in cooking.

Citrus Fruits

a. Citrus fruits—which include oranges, lemons, and grapefruits—are known for having a high acidic content, which can cause heartburn and acid reflux in people who have Barrett's oesophagus. Citrus fruit consumption has the ability to lower stomach pH, which may relax the LES and raise the risk of gastric reflux into the oesophagus.

b. Research studies have clarified the relationship between eating citrus fruits and aggravated acid reflux symptoms, highlighting the need for those with Barrett's oesophagus to consume these fruits with caution. Furthermore, citrus fruits' high vitamin C content, although advantageous in other situations, might aggravate and cause discomfort in the oesophagus of those who are managing Barrett's oesophagus.

c. : Citrus fruits have been shown in research studies and patient testimonials to exacerbate symptoms of acid reflux and heartburn in people with Barrett's oesophagus. Patients who have reduced or stopped eating citrus fruits have attested to a noticeable improvement in esophageal comfort and symptom control.

d. Practical Applications: To lessen the risk of aggravating acid reflux and esophageal irritation, replacing citrus fruits with less acidic options like apples, pears, and bananas can be a safer and more esophageal-friendly option.

Carbonated Beverages

a. Carbon dioxide, which is included in carbonated drinks like sodas and fizzy drinks, can expand the stomach and put pressure on the LES, causing it to relax and making the stomach more likely to reflux food into the oesophagus. For those who have Barrett's oesophagus, the rush of acidic gastric contents into the oesophagus can cause or worsen symptoms of acid reflux and heartburn.

b. Clinical studies have highlighted the link between the consumption of carbonated beverages and an increased risk of acid reflux episodes, thus those who are managing Barrett's oesophagus should be cautious when consuming them. Furthermore, obesity and weight gain are recognised risk factors for the advancement of Barrett's oesophagus, and they can be exacerbated by the high sugar content in many carbonated beverages.

c. : Clinical study data as well as patient testimonials have repeatedly demonstrated how carbonated drinks exacerbate acid reflux symptoms in people with Barrett's oesophagus. Patient testimonials describing a discernible improvement in esophageal comfort and symptom management have been obtained from individuals who have cut back or stopped drinking carbonated beverages.

d. Practical Applications: Choosing non-carbonated, non-acidic substitutes like water, diluted fruit juices, or herbal teas can provide a more esophageally-friendly option, reducing the risk of aggravating esophageal irritation and acid reflux.

High-fat Foods

a. Foods high in fat, especially those high in saturated and trans fats, can cause a delay in the emptying of the stomach, which increases the risk of gastric reflux into the oesophagus and prolongs stomach distension. High-fat meal consumption has the potential to relax the LES, which can exacerbate esophageal discomfort in Barrett's esophagitis patients and cause reflux of acidic stomach contents.

b. Studies have demonstrated the link between eating a diet high in fat and having more acid reflux episodes, which may exacerbate esophageal inflammation and the severity of symptoms in those with Barrett's oesophagus. Furthermore, obesity and weight gain are recognised risk factors for the advancement of Barrett's oesophagus, and they can be exacerbated by the high calorie content of high-fat diets.

c. : Clinical studies and patient reports have repeatedly demonstrated how high-fat diets exacerbate acid reflux symptoms in people with Barrett's oesophagus. Patients who have reduced or stopped eating meals high in fat have reported a noticeable improvement in symptom management and esophageal comfort.

d. Practical Applications: Leaner options, such lean meats, low-fat dairy products, and healthy fats, can offer a more esophageally-friendly option, lowering the risk of aggravating esophageal discomfort and acid reflux.

Processed and Fried Foods

a. Foods that are processed or fried, due to their high content of harmful fats, additives, and preservatives, can worsen heartburn and acid reflux symptoms in those who have Barrett's oesophagus. Eating these meals may cause the LES to relax, delay the emptying of the stomach, and raise the risk of gastric reflux into the oesophagus, which may worsen esophageal discomfort.

b. Clinical studies have indicated a correlation between the intake of processed and fried meals and a higher frequency of acid reflux episodes; therefore, those who are managing Barrett's oesophagus should be cautious while consuming these items. Furthermore, these foods' low nutritional value and high calorie content can lead to weight gain and obesity, which are recognised risk factors for the advancement of Barrett's oesophagus.

c. : Research has shown that eating processed and fried meals increases the frequency of acid reflux episodes; therefore, those who are managing Barrett's oesophagus should limit their intake of these items. Moreover, these foods' high calorie content and poor nutritional value might cause weight gain and obesity, which are recognised risk factors for the advancement of Barrett's oesophagus.

d. Practical Applications: A more esophageally-friendly option can be obtained by selecting complete, unprocessed alternatives and using healthy cooking techniques, like baking, grilling, or steaming. This lowers the risk of escalating acid reflux and esophageal discomfort.

:

A key element of an integrated approach to esophageal health is the careful evaluation of foods to avoid in the management of Barrett's oesophagus. As we continue to explore the nuances of dietary management, it is clear that careful food selection has a major impact on both the intensity of symptoms and the general health of the oesophagus. We will continue to explore the many approaches to maximising esophageal health in the upcoming chapters, emphasising the critical role that dietary treatments play in this process.

Meal Planning and Preparation Tips

Introduction:

The nuances of meal planning and preparation are crucial to maintaining adherence to a diet that is Barrett's-friendly when it comes to the careful management of Barrett's oesophagus. This chapter aims to offer a thorough manual to help people create and carry out meal plans that comply with dietary guidelines for Barrett's oesophagus management. This chapter attempts to walk readers through each step of the methodical road map of actions and procedures that must be followed in order to accomplish the particular goal of effective meal planning and preparation.

This chapter's main goal is to provide readers with the information and useful skills they need to create Barrett's-friendly menus and carry out efficient food preparation techniques. Reaching this objective will enable readers to incorporate dietary changes that support Barrett's oesophagus management into their everyday routines.

Prior to beginning the process of meal planning and preparation for the treatment of Barrett's oesophagus, it is necessary to become acquainted with the following requirements:

1. a thorough awareness of the dietary guidelines for people with Barrett's oesophagus, including what foods to avoid and what is best for esophageal health.

2. availability of a wide range of Barrett's-friendly foods, such as fruits, vegetables, lean meats, and whole grains.

3. Basic cooking abilities, including cutting, sautéing, and baking, can make Barrett's-friendly dishes easier to prepare.

4. Meal planning tools to make meal preparation easier, include a weekly calendar, grocery list, and portion control recommendations.

Developing Barrett's-friendly menus and putting good food preparation techniques into practise involve a number of crucial tasks, such as:

1. Understanding Dietary Guidelines: Learning about the foods that are good for the health of the oesophagus and what foods are recommended for people with Barrett's oesophagus.

2. Meal Planning: putting up a planned menu that takes into account dietary limitations and preferences while including Barrett's-friendly items.

3. Ingredient Selection: selecting premium, fresh products that support esophageal health and correspond with Barrett's oesophagus dietary guidelines.

4. Culinary Techniques: use appropriate cooking techniques, such as grilling, baking, and steaming, to make wholesome, tasty meals that are Barrett's-friendly.

5. Portion Control: following portion control tips to guarantee that meals are sized and balanced according to dietary rules.

Understanding Dietary Guidelines:

It is essential to familiarise oneself with the dietary rules for Barrett's oesophagus before beginning meal planning and preparation. This means understanding the list of items to stay away from, as explained in the previous chapter, and figuring out substitute elements that are good for the health of your oesophagus. Making educated decisions during meal planning and preparation also requires understanding the nutritional makeup of Barrett's-friendly foods, including their fibre content, vitamin and mineral profiles, and possible effects on esophageal health.

Meal Planning:

Meal planning for Barrett's oesophagus management is organising meals and snacks into a set timetable that complies with nutritional guidelines. This includes:

- Weekly Meal Plans: creating a detailed weekly plan that includes the meals and snacks for every day and includes a wide variety of Barrett's-friendly foods, such as fruits, vegetables, whole grains, and lean proteins.

- Consideration of Dietary Preferences and Restrictions: To ensure that meals are both appropriate and pleasant, meal plans can be customised to satisfy particular dietary preferences, such as vegetarian or gluten-free diets, as well as constraints, such lactose intolerance or allergies.

- Balance and Variety: Aiming for a diverse range of food groups and a balance of macronutrients in every meal, including healthy fats, carbs, proteins, and a range of vitamins and minerals to promote esophageal health and overall health.

Ingredient Selection:

The foundation of a successful meal prep is the selection of premium, Barrett's-friendly ingredients. This includes:

- Fresh and Nutrient-Dense Ingredients: Choosing lean proteins, healthy grains, and fresh produce can guarantee that meals are high in vital nutrients and support esophageal health.

- Reading Labels: Examining food labels closely in order to spot possible triggers or undesirable substances (such processed, acidic, or high-fat foods), then basing choices on this knowledge.

- Culinary Adaptations: Using appropriate substitutes for elements that are typically avoided in the treatment of Barrett's oesophagus, such as low-fat dairy products to reduce the escalation of esophageal symptoms and the use of non-citrus-based acids in marinades or sauces.

Culinary Techniques:

The creation of foods that are suitable for Barrett's requires the application of certain cooking techniques. This includes:

- Healthy Cooking Methods: Using cooking methods like baking, grilling, and steaming that reduce the amount of added fats and oils, maintain the nutritional value of the ingredients, and reduce the chance of making esophageal discomfort worse.

- Flavor Enhancements: investigating different ways to add taste to food—like herbs, spices, and aromatics—instead of depending on substances that can be harmful to the health of the oesophagus.

- Texture Modification: modifying cooking methods to produce desired textures; for example, using pureed or finely chopped food to reduce esophageal irritation and make swallowing easier.

Portion Control:

To guarantee that meals are properly sized and balanced in compliance with nutritional requirements, portion control standards must be followed. This includes:

- Utilizing Measuring Tools: Portion control, measuring cups, and scales are tools that help portion meals and snacks precisely, which reduces overindulgence and raises awareness of portion sizes.

- Balancing Macronutrients: making an effort to balance the macronutrients—carbs, proteins, and fats—in each meal in order to promote esophageal health and general health.

- Mindful Eating Practices: Developing awareness when eating to appreciate tastes, textures, and scents as well as to help foods that are Barrett's-friendly digest and be enjoyed to the fullest.

- Collaborative Meal Planning: Creating meals together with family members or caregivers can help to create a welcoming atmosphere and make it easier to incorporate Barrett's-friendly cuisine into family mealtimes.

- Label Analysis: When choosing packaged or processed foods, it might be helpful to carefully read food labels in order to detect potential triggers and make well-informed decisions about the compatibility of ingredients.

- Culinary Creativity: Barrett's-friendly meal plans can be made more exciting and diverse by embracing culinary creativity and experimenting with new dishes and ingredients. This will make managing Barrett's oesophagus through diet fun and sustainable.

- Mindful Consumption: Eating mindfully can lessen the risk of esophageal discomfort and improve healthy digestion. This includes eating slowly, digesting food completely, and maintaining a calm posture while eating.

The following signs can be used to confirm that successful meal planning and preparation procedures have been implemented:

- Adherence to Dietary Recommendations: Meal plans and prepared meals should be in line with the dietary guidelines for Barrett's oesophagus, which include avoiding trigger foods and include components that are favourable to the oesophagus.

- Symptom Management: noticing a reduction in the intensity of symptoms and an improvement in esophageal comfort after Barrett's-friendly meal plans and preparation techniques were put into practise, as reported by self-evaluation and consultation with medical professionals.

- Sustained Compliance: displaying consistent adherence to Barrett's-friendly meal plans and preparation techniques over a long period of time, a sign of the incorporation of dietary adjustments into daily routines and way of life.

If difficulties or obstacles arise when organising meals and getting ready for Barrett's oesophagus care, the following options could be taken into consideration:

- Consultation with Healthcare Providers: requesting advice from medical professionals, such as gastroenterologists and certified dietitians, in order to address certain dietary issues and receive individualised suggestions catered to individual requirements.

- Culinary Adaptations: investigating other culinary modifications to satisfy particular dietary requirements and enhance dish palatability, such as altering textures or using different cooking techniques.

- Continuous Education: maintaining current knowledge of new culinary methods, substitute ingredients, and esophageal health studies in addition to participating in continuing education and awareness-raising addressing the dietary management of Barrett's oesophagus.

:

A key component of complete esophageal health management is the careful planning and preparation of Barrett's-friendly meals, which assist patients on their path to better symptom control and general well-being. The careful selection of ingredients and cooking methods can have a substantial impact on esophageal comfort and quality of life as we delve deeper into the nuances of dietary therapies for Barrett's oesophagus. We will go more into the many approaches of maximising esophageal health in the upcoming chapters, emphasising the critical role that dietary treatments play in this life-changing process.

Understanding Nutrition Labels

Comprehending nutrition labels is an essential ability for people who want to make educated food decisions. It is the starting point for understanding the nutritional makeup of food items, allowing customers to identify vital nutrients, possible allergies, and additives that could be harmful to their health. Therefore, encouraging a thoughtful approach to food selection and consumption requires a knowledge of deciphering nutrition labels.

To facilitate a comprehensive understanding of nutrition labels, the following key terms are essential for elucidation:

1. Serving Size
2. Calories
3. Macronutrients (Protein, Carbohydrates, and Fats)
4. Fiber
5. Added Sugars
6. Sodium
7. Ingredients List
8. Daily Values

1. The serving size lists the number of servings in the package as well as the suggested portion of the product to be taken at one time. Comprehending serving sizes is essential to properly evaluating the food product's nutritional value in respect to one's dietary needs.

2. The amount of energy that a serving of a food product contains is measured in calories. The number of calories in each serving must be taken into account while controlling total energy consumption and selecting a balanced diet.

3. An appropriate diet must include macronutrients. Carbs give you energy, proteins are necessary for tissue growth and repair, and fats are necessary for hormone regulation and nutrient absorption. Creating a diet that is nutritionally sound requires an understanding of the quantity and quality of macronutrients in food products.

4. A non-digestible carbohydrate that aids in satiety and digestive health is fibre. Foods rich in fibre improve general health and help control blood sugar and cholesterol levels.

5. Sugars added during processing or preparation are known as added sugars. Those who want to control their total sugar intake and minimise their consumption of refined sugars must keep an eye out for added sugars.

6. The sodium level of a food item indicates how much salt is in it. It is imperative for those with certain health concerns, such hypertension or cardiovascular disorders, to keep an eye on their sodium consumption.

7. The ingredients list, which is presented in descending order of weight predominance, offers a thorough inventory of all the substances utilised in the manufacturing of the food product. 8. Daily Values are benchmarks set by health authorities to help customers evaluate a food product's nutritional value in relation to a daily diet. Knowing the components list is essential for spotting any allergies or unwanted chemicals. They serve as a standard for assessing the nutritional sufficiency of a serving of the food product and are stated as percentages.

8. Understanding these essential phrases is comparable to using a map. Understanding nutrition labels provides people with the knowledge and skills necessary to navigate the nutritional landscape of food products, much as how one uses a map to comprehend the terrain, locate landmarks, and get to their destination. It gives them the ability to make wise choices, avoid dietary pitfalls, and set themselves up for optimum health and wellbeing.

When people start this adventure of learning how to read nutrition labels, they are like explorers with the skills to figure out what foods contain nutritionally, much like how you read a map's symbols and legends. This analogy emphasises how crucial it is to comprehend nutrition labels as a prerequisite knowledge before setting out on an informed and health-conscious food journey.

-

In addition to the introduction, I have included a list of key terminology, their explanations, and connections between these phrases and ideas from everyday life. Should I move on to the following part now?

Supplements and Barrett's Oesophagus

The disorder known as Barrett's Oesophagus is typified by aberrant cellular alterations in the lower part of the oesophagus, frequently brought on by persistent acid reflux. Because of its link to a higher risk of developing oesophageal cancer, this condition is very concerning. It can be difficult for patients with Barrett's oesophagus to manage their illness in order to stop it from getting worse and reduce the hazards involved. The therapy of Barrett's oesophagus is mostly dependent on lifestyle changes and traditional medical therapies, however there is reason to be cautious about the possible contribution of dietary supplements to this management.

Developing comprehensive therapies that address the underlying pathological alterations in the oesophageal tissue is one of the main challenges in addressing Barrett's Oesophagus. Furthermore, a multimodal approach to care is required due to the possibility of the illness progressing to a more advanced stage, such as dysplasia or adenocarcinoma. While lifestyle modifications and proton pump inhibitors are effective conventional therapy methods, there is still a lack of knowledge on the possible significance of dietary supplements in enhancing these approaches.

If the special problems associated with Barrett's oesophagus are not addressed, the disease may worsen and the risk of oesophageal cancer may rise. Poor treatment can also result in discomfort and acid reflux symptoms that don't go away, which lowers the quality of life for those who have this illness. As a result, it is critical to investigate and comprehend the possible repercussions of ignoring dietary supplements when managing Barrett's oesophagus.

Given the intricate nature of managing Barrett's oesophagus, adding carefully chosen dietary supplements could be a viable way to provide all-encompassing support. Through the utilisation of targeted supplements, patients with Barrett's Oesophagus may enhance conventional therapy methods and target underlying pathophysiological mechanisms, ultimately contributing to a more comprehensive care plan.

A methodical strategy is necessary for the incorporation of dietary supplements into the management of Barrett's oesophagus. This procedure includes determining which particular supplements have benefits supported by research, taking into account any possible drug interactions, and creating customised dosage schedules. To guarantee the safe and efficient integration of dietary supplements into the overall treatment plan, cooperation with healthcare practitioners and ongoing monitoring are also crucial.

Research examining the possible influence of dietary supplements on the management of Barrett's oesophagus has yielded encouraging results. Some supplements, for example, have demonstrated antioxidant and anti-inflammatory qualities as well as the capacity to alter cellular mechanisms linked to the advancement of Barrett's oesophagus. Analyzing these historical and anticipated results makes it clear that the deliberate application of dietary supplements has substantial promise for improving the overall treatment of this illness.

Although dietary supplements provide an additional means of managing Barrett's oesophagus, it is important to recognise that there are other options. Novel medicinal interventions, specific lifestyle changes, or newly developed therapy modalities are a few examples of these. Assessing these possibilities yields a thorough comprehension of the diverse array of choices accessible to persons managing the intricacies of Barrett's oesophagus.

We will discuss the particular dietary supplements that show promise for Barrett's oesophagus therapy in the sections that follow. The potential advantages, modes of action, and factors to be taken into account when incorporating each supplement into a customised treatment plan will all be covered in detail, offering a thorough resource for patients and medical professionals looking to maximise the management of Barrett's oesophagus.

-

The particular dietary supplements that have demonstrated promise in the treatment of Barrett's oesophagus will be discussed in more detail in the next section. We will look closely at these supplements, covering their modes of action, dosage requirements, and data pertaining to their ability to maintain oesophageal health.

Recipes for Healing

This section's objective is to offer a wide range of mouthwatering dishes that not only fit the dietary requirements required to manage Barrett's Oesophagus but are also delectable. With a wide range of nutrient-dense and Barrett's-friendly dishes, this all-inclusive resource seeks to encourage wholesome and pleasurable eating habits specific to those who suffer from this illness.

The recipes found in this area can be made using readily available items and are intended to be enjoyed by a broad range of cooks. It is advised to keep a basic kitchen equipped with gadgets and culinary tools. To make sure that the components in these recipes comply with certain dietary requirements or considerations, it is also advisable to speak with medical professionals or trained dietitians.

This section's recipes, which include breakfast alternatives, main meals, side dishes, and desserts, span a variety of culinary genres. Every dish has been carefully designed to maximise nutritious content and reduce any possible causes of acid reflux. These recipes attempt to improve treatment of Barrett's oesophagus and promote overall wellness by utilising a variety of whole foods, herbs, and spices.

1. - Nutritious Smoothie Bowl: a cool concoction of almond milk, spinach, and mixed berries garnished with sliced almonds and chia seeds. This meal is easy on the stomach and offers a high-fiber, antioxidant-rich breakfast.

- Oatmeal with Cinnamon and Fresh Fruit: A hearty and satisfying breakfast choice made with vibrant fresh fruit, whole rolled oats, and a dash of cinnamon. This dish makes a filling, high-fiber breakfast.

2. - Baked Lemon Herb Chicken: Flavorful marinated chicken breasts roasted to perfection with a zingy mixture of lemon juice, garlic, and fresh herbs. This tasty and well-balanced supper is served with a side of steamed veggies and a protein-rich entrée.

- Quinoa and Vegetable Stir-Fry: A bright stir-fry with tofu, colourful bell peppers, snap peas, and fluffy quinoa seasoned with a savoury but light sauce. This vegan recipe offers important nutrients and a source of protein.

3. - Mashed Sweet Potatoes with Herbs: Sweet potatoes mashed to a creamy consistency with a dash of olive oil and aromatic herbs. Packed with vitamins and minerals, this hearty side dish supports general health and wellbeing.

- Steamed Asparagus with Lemon Zest: Steamed fresh asparagus spears with a dash of lemon zest for extra flavour. This understated yet sophisticated side dish provides vital nutrients and a taste explosion.

4. - Berry and Yogurt Parfait: Layers of crunchy granola, juicy berries, and tart Greek yoghurt combine to make a tasty and healthy dessert or snack. This recipe offers just the right amount of sweetness and texture without sacrificing choices that are good for you.

- Poached Pears with Cinnamon: Perfectly ripe pears poached in a fragrant syrup laced with cinnamon, creating a naturally sweet and tender treat. This sophisticated dish provides a fulfilling mealtime finish without taxing the digestive tract.

- The use of fresh, whole ingredients should be prioritised when making these recipes, and processed or highly seasoned foods should be avoided as they may aggravate Barrett's oesophagus symptoms.

- Combining different hues and textures into meals not only makes them seem better, but it also guarantees that the nutrients being consumed are varied, which is good for your health in general.

- When choosing and adjusting recipes, it's critical to take into account each person's sensitivities and preferences. You should also adjust portion sizes to suit individual dietary needs.

- Even though these recipes are meant to be Barrett's-friendly, it's crucial for people to keep an eye on how they personally react to various components and modify their meal plans accordingly.

In order to confirm that these recipes are being successfully followed, people are advised to keep a food journal in which they record what they eat and any symptoms that may arise. Furthermore, regular discussions with medical professionals or licenced dietitians can offer insightful information on how these recipes affect personal management techniques.

If there are any foods or cooking methods that people with Barrett's oesophagus find difficult to use, it is advisable to look into substitutes that meet certain dietary needs. Individual sensitivities can be accommodated by making substitutions, such as switching to lower-acid versions of some foods or using marinades without citrus.

Through the inclusion of these Barrett's-friendly recipes in daily meal planning, patients can adopt a comprehensive approach to controlling their disease while indulging in a varied and satisfying gastronomic experience.

-

In the next section, we will discuss meal planning and nutritional issues unique to people with Barrett's oesophagus, providing helpful advice for developing a balanced and health-promoting eating pattern.

Holistic Approaches to Management

The Role of Stress Reduction

The Role of Stress Reduction in Managing Barrett's Esophagus

Introduction

The aberrant alterations in the lower esophageal cells that characterise Barrett's oesophagus are frequently brought on by chronic gastroesophageal reflux disease (GERD). Barrett's oesophagus is managed using a multimodal strategy that includes behavioural, psychological, and medicinal therapies. An important and sometimes disregarded element in the development and treatment of Barrett's oesophagus is stress. The purpose of this chapter is to examine how stress affects Barrett's oesophagus and to suggest ways to reduce stress as a crucial component of the overall care strategy.

Define the Problem

It has been demonstrated that stress, especially prolonged stress, can make a number of gastrointestinal disorders worse, including GERD, which is a significant risk factor for the development of Barrett's oesophagus. Stress hormones like cortisol and adrenaline are released when people are under stress because the body naturally reacts to stress by going into heightened awareness. These physiological changes have the potential to worsen GERD symptoms and advance Barrett's oesophagus by increasing the generation of gastric acid, delaying gastric emptying, and altering gastrointestinal motility.

People with Barrett's oesophagus may experience a vicious cycle of worsening symptoms, lowering quality of life, and maybe even accelerating the disease's progression if stress is not adequately handled. According to studies, those with Barrett's oesophagus who are under a lot of stress are more prone to develop esophageal dysmotility, greater exposure to esophageal acid, and severe GERD symptoms. Chronic stress has also been linked to increased inflammation, weakened mucosal defence systems, and a compromised immune system, all of which can worsen the underlying pathophysiology of Barrett's oesophagus.

Since stress has a major effect on Barrett's oesophagus, it is essential to include stress management strategies in the treatment strategy. The physiological and psychological impacts of stress may be lessened by mind-body therapies like mindfulness-based stress reduction (MBSR), cognitive-behavioral therapy (CBT), and relaxation methods. By modifying the body's stress response, encouraging emotional control, and improving coping mechanisms, these methods may lessen the negative effects of stress on Barrett's oesophagus.

Detail the Implementation

Applying stress-reduction strategies requires a customised, all-encompassing strategy that takes into account each person's unique stressors, coping strategies, and lifestyle choices. Barrett's oesophagus management necessitates a multidisciplinary approach comprising medical specialists such as gastroenterologists, psychologists, and nutritionists in order to incorporate stress reduction. Individualized stress management programmes that include regular therapy sessions, mindfulness training, food changes, and lifestyle improvements to reduce stresses can be beneficial for patients.

Research indicates that integrating stress-reduction strategies into the treatment of gastrointestinal disorders can result in positive effects. Research has indicated that participants in stress reduction therapies report significantly better overall well-being, fewer episodes of esophageal acid exposure, and GERD symptoms. Additionally, including stress-reduction strategies has demonstrated promise in regulating immunological response, decreasing inflammatory response, and enhancing mucosal integrity—all of which are important for Barrett's oesophagus care.

While addressing stress-related Barrett's esophagitis aggravation requires the use of stress reduction approaches, it's vital to recognise that pharmacological therapies may be necessary in some circumstances. The prudent use of anxiolytic or antidepressant medications, under the supervision of a psychiatrist or mental health professional, may be taken into consideration as an adjunct to non-pharmacological stress reduction strategies for individuals experiencing severe exacerbation of stress-related symptoms. Nonetheless, pharmacotherapy should only be used after thorough evaluation and individualised for each patient's unique needs, with close monitoring for any possible side effects and combinations with other medications.

Conclusion

Finally, stress is an important variable that might affect how Barrett's oesophagus develops and is managed. It appears that integrating stress-reduction strategies into the overall care plan will help lessen the negative impact of stress on the illness. Healthcare professionals can provide a more comprehensive strategy to managing Barrett's oesophagus by addressing stress as a crucial component. This approach addresses not only the physical symptoms of the disease but also the psychological and emotional well-being of individuals. In the future, more investigation and clinical application of stress-reduction techniques are necessary to enhance Barrett's oesophagus therapy and enhance patient outcomes.

Beneficial Exercises for Barrett's Patients

Exercise is very important for Barrett's oesophagus management since it has several advantages that are both psychologically and physically beneficial. The exercises listed below have been carefully chosen to offer safe and helpful options for those who have Barrett's oesophagus. The goals of these exercises are to promote overall well-being, lower stress levels, and improve gastrointestinal function.

a. Exercising at a moderate level, such cycling, swimming, or brisk walking, has several benefits for people who have Barrett's oesophagus. These exercises help to manage weight, strengthen respiratory health, and improve cardiovascular health—all of which are critical components of the condition's overall care. Furthermore, it has been demonstrated that aerobic exercise reduces tension and anxiety, providing psychological advantages that may enhance the quality of life for those who have Barrett's oesophagus.

b. Yoga and Tai Chi are becoming more well-known for their all-encompassing approach to wellness, which includes physical postures, breathing exercises, and meditation. These mind-body exercises provide a gentle yet efficient way to increase relaxation, lower stress levels, and improve flexibility for those with Barrett's oesophagus. Tai Chi's flowing, soft movements and yoga's attentive, regulated poses are beneficial supplements to any fitness plan since they can improve both emotional and gastrointestinal health.

c. Strength training activities, including bodyweight exercises or resistance band workouts, can improve bone density, muscular endurance, and strength—all of which are important for managing Barrett's oesophagus. Strength training has also been linked to better weight control and metabolic health, which may be advantageous for people trying to manage comorbidities like obesity or metabolic syndrome. For those with Barrett's oesophagus, stressing correct technique and deliberate breathing during strength training sessions can further improve the safety and effectiveness of these activities.

d. It may be possible to reduce the symptoms of Barrett's oesophagus by doing breathing exercises like pursed lip breathing or diaphragmatic breathing. The primary goals of these exercises are to improve breathing, induce relaxation, and lessen stress—all of which can have a significant impact on the quality of life for those who suffer from the illness. Breathing exercises are a useful tool for people with Barrett's oesophagus because they help them become more conscious of their breath, which may help lessen the negative effects of stress and anxiety on their digestive system.

e. For people with Barrett's oesophagus, flexibility exercises such as light stretching regimens and mobility drills are quite beneficial. These exercises are designed to increase overall flexibility, release tension in the muscles, and increase range of motion. These benefits can all lead to better posture, less discomfort, and enhanced physical function. Furthermore, adding flexibility training to the exercise routine can act as a type of mindful movement, encouraging a state of peace and relaxation that can help Barrett's oesophagus patients manage their stress.

Studies have demonstrated the beneficial effects of exercise on digestive health, and there is evidence to support the idea that regular exercise can lessen the likelihood of gastroesophageal reflux and alleviate Barrett's oesophagus symptoms. Testimonials from people with Barrett's oesophagus who have made exercise a regular part of their routine frequently highlight the feelings of empowerment, better moods, and increased physical function that come with leading an active lifestyle.

Including these activities in the regimen of people with Barrett's oesophagus requires a customised approach based on the patient's medical history, degree of fitness, and personal preferences. Developing specialised exercise regimens that put safety, enjoyment, and adherence first can be made easier by collaborating with healthcare professionals like physiotherapists or exercise specialists. Moreover, integrating these activities into everyday life—whether through focused training sessions or integrated mobility throughout the day—can result in noticeable advantages for those attempting to manage Barrett's oesophagus in its entirety.

By include these exercises in the Barrett's oesophagus treatment plan, a comprehensive strategy that takes into account both the physical and psychological aspects of the illness is provided. Through promoting a more comprehensive comprehension of the advantages and pragmatic aspects linked to every exercise, people with Barrett's oesophagus can make well-informed choices regarding the incorporation of physical activity into their everyday routines, ultimately leading to enhanced quality of life.

Mindfulness and Meditation Practices

The integration of mindfulness and meditation techniques is crucial for the comprehensive care of Barrett's oesophagus. Through these meditative practises, people can develop emotional resilience, lower their stress levels, and become more acutely aware of their bodily and mental health. People can begin a life-changing journey that not only enhances medical interventions but also gives them the ability to take an active role in their own care by incorporating mindfulness and meditation into their daily routine. The purpose of this chapter is to clarify the fundamentals of mindfulness and meditation, as well as their possible advantages when it comes to Barrett's oesophagus and offer helpful advice on how to include them in an all-encompassing treatment strategy.

This chapter aims to give the reader a thorough understanding of mindfulness and meditation techniques, explaining how they may help with Barrett's oesophagus management and offering helpful advice on how to put them into practise.

There aren't many requirements to practise mindfulness and meditation. The main prerequisites are a place that is calm and distraction-free as well as a willingness to dedicate time for regular practise. Even while they are not necessary, people may find it helpful to use tools like yoga mats, meditation pillows, or apps to enhance their practise.

Barrett's oesophagus management with mindfulness and meditation incorporates a multimodal approach to improve emotional health, lower stress levels, and develop a stronger bond between the mind and body. In order to promote general health and well-being, this approach entails gradually cultivating mindfulness, creating a variety of meditation practises, and incorporating them into daily life.

a. Originating in contemplative traditions like Buddhism, mindfulness entails the deliberate practise of cultivating present-moment awareness without passing judgement. With an open mind and acceptance, this practise invites people to examine their ideas, feelings, and physical experiences. Barrett's oesophagus sufferers can become more attuned to their bodies' cues through mindfulness, which can help them react to physical pain or emotional stress more calmly and mindfully.

b. There is a wide range of meditation practises, each with a specific function in fostering emotional equilibrium, mental clarity, and relaxation. People can practise a variety of techniques to develop a stronger sense of inner peace and self-awareness, including guided meditation, breath-focused meditation, loving-kindness meditation, and body scan meditation. With the help of these methods, people can learn how to control their stress levels, anxiety, and the psychological effects of having Barrett's oesophagus.

c. Incorporating moments of present and concentration into everyday activities, including eating, walking, or performing household chores, is one way that people might practise mindfulness. For example, mindful eating promotes people to enjoy every mouthful, pay attention to signs of hunger and fullness, and form a positive relationship with food. This can be especially helpful for people who need to adjust their diet because of Barrett's oesophagus.

d. Maintaining consistency is essential to gaining from mindfulness and meditation. It is recommended that people set aside time on a regular basis for their practise, which can take the shape of guided meditation, formal sitting meditation, or simply incorporating mindful moments into everyday activities. By making this time, people can cultivate emotional well-being, handle stress, and nourish their inner resilience.

- Begin with Short Sessions: Starting with short sessions, like five to ten minutes, can enable those who are new to mindfulness and meditation gradually become accustomed to the practise without becoming overwhelmed.

- Embrace Non-Judgment: People who practise mindfulness are more inclined to observe their experiences objectively. Adopting a non-judgmental viewpoint can help people become more self-compassionate and less critical of themselves, which is especially important for those who are juggling the demands of managing a chronic illness.

- Seek Guided Resources: By giving people organised direction and encouraging words, guided meditation tools like audio recordings and apps can be a great help to people in their practise.

- Be Patient and Persistent: The process of developing awareness and making meditation a regular part of one's life happens gradually. The development of a contemplative practise that is both enriching and durable requires the virtues of patience and endurance.

The incorporation of mindfulness and meditation practises into the treatment of Barrett's oesophagus can be demonstrated by the measurable improvement in emotional well-being, a decrease in stress, and an increased ability to deal with the difficulties brought on by the condition with more composure and resilience.

If people find it difficult to stick with a regular meditation routine or find that their thoughts are taking over during the practise, it might be helpful to speak with mindfulness instructors, meditation teachers, or mental health specialists for individualised advice and support.

People with Barrett's oesophagus can greatly benefit from mindfulness and meditation activities in terms of fostering their mental and physical well-being. Through the adoption of mindfulness principles, experimentation with various meditation techniques, and integration of these practises into daily life, individuals can initiate a profound journey that enhances their ability to manage the intricacies of their health with increased resilience, composure, and self-awareness. A holistic strategy that recognises the interdependence of body, mind, and spirit is highlighted by the incorporation of mindfulness and meditation into the all-encompassing management of

Barrett's oesophagus. This promotes a strong sense of empowerment in the face of health obstacles.

The Power of Sleep and Rest

Barrett's oesophagus requires an all-encompassing approach to therapy, one that includes not only dietary and pharmacological changes but also the critical role that rest and sleep play. A basic physiological necessity, sleep is essential for general health, wellbeing, and sickness recovery. But the importance of getting enough sleep and the influence of quiet times on managing Barrett's oesophagus are frequently disregarded. The purpose of this chapter is to clarify the significance of sleep and rest in relation to Barrett's oesophagus management. It does this by describing the possible negative effects of sleep deprivation and insufficient rest and by suggesting workable ways to improve sleep quality and schedule rest periods.

The main problem here is the widespread ignorance of how important relaxation and sleep are to the overall care of Barrett's oesophagus. Modern civilization is rife with sleep deprivation and low quality sleep, with people frequently putting job, social obligations, and screen time ahead of getting enough sleep. In the case of Barrett's oesophagus, inadequate sleep can worsen symptoms, impede the healing process, and impair general wellbeing, making management extremely difficult.

The ramifications of insufficient sleep and rest for people diagnosed with Barrett's oesophagus are complex. In the context of Barrett's oesophagus, physiologically speaking, sleep deprivation can hinder tissue healing, weaken the body's ability to manage inflammation, and alter the immune system. Furthermore, prolonged sleep deprivation and poor sleep quality can worsen anxiety, despair, and stress, which can have a detrimental effect on one's emotional health and general quality of life.

It is critical to stress the need of prioritising sleep and putting mechanisms in place to maximise the quality of sleep in order to address the issue of insufficient rest and sleep in the context of managing Barrett's oesophagus. People can improve their general health and help manage Barrett's oesophagus more effectively by creating an atmosphere that encourages restful sleep and incorporating intervals of rest into everyday activities.

a. Promoting peaceful sleep requires creating a sleep-friendly environment. This include keeping the temperature in the room at a comfortable level, reducing light and noise disruptions, and making sure the sleeping surface is pleasant with a supportive mattress and appropriate pillows. Furthermore, people can profit by developing a pre-sleep pattern that instructs the body and mind to enter a relaxed state. Examples of such routines include doing relaxing exercises or relaxing hobbies before bed.

b. Optimizing sleep quality requires adherence to excellent sleep hygiene practises. This entails keeping regular wake-up and sleep schedules, abstaining from stimulants like caffeine and electronics near to bedtime, and getting regular exercise to encourage sound sleep. Furthermore, it is advised that people avoid consuming large meals and alcohol right before bed because they can interfere with sleep cycles and exacerbate symptoms of Barrett's oesophagus.

c. Apart from maximising nocturnal sleep, incorporating intervals of relaxation into everyday schedules might offer significant chances for unwinding and revitalization. People can gain by taking little naps or moments of relaxation during the day, such as mindfulness activities, deep breathing techniques, or light stretching. These downtimes have the potential to reduce stress, enhance emotional health, and support equilibrium and renewal.

Barrett's oesophagus can be effectively managed by optimising the quality of sleep and scheduling rest intervals into daily routines, according to the evidence recommending their use. Better sleep has been linked to a stronger immune system, less inflammation, and general improvements in both physical and mental health. Furthermore, those who place a high priority on getting enough sleep and rest report being better able to handle the difficulties of having Barrett's oesophagus, which enables them to take a more proactive and in charge attitude to their health.

Although the above-mentioned strategies provide a solid basis for optimising sleep and rest within the context of managing Barrett's oesophagus, people may find it helpful to experiment with other methods like relaxation therapies or cognitive-behavioral interventions for sleep, or to seek professional advice from healthcare providers or sleep specialists to address specific sleep-related issues.

In summary, an essential component of the all-encompassing care of Barrett's oesophagus is the incorporation of sleep optimization techniques and the scheduling of rest periods into everyday activities. Through addressing the vital role that rest and sleep play in health and healing, people can improve their general health, lessen the negative effects of stress and inflammation, and actively participate in the management of Barrett's oesophagus. Accepting the importance of rest and sleep emphasises a holistic strategy that recognises the connection between psychological and physiological elements, resulting in a deep sense of empowerment in managing the complexities of health issues.

Integrative Medicine Options

The combination of integrative medicine approaches alongside conventional treatment has tremendous potential in the holistic care of Barrett's oesophagus. These alternative therapies include a wide range of therapy modalities that can improve the general health of patients with Barrett's oesophagus when paired with traditional medical care. The essential integrative medicine alternatives listed below can help manage Barrett's oesophagus holistically by providing information about their mechanisms, evidence-based backing, and useful uses.

a. A key component of Barrett's oesophagus management is nutritional therapy, which focuses on dietary changes that promote gastrointestinal health and reduce reflux symptoms. Stressing the importance of eating complete foods—especially those high in fibre and antioxidants—can reduce inflammation and improve digestive health. Furthermore, it has been demonstrated that including particular nutrients in the diet, like zinc and glutamine, helps to maintain esophageal integrity and promote mucosal repair. There is evidence that nutritional therapy can help manage Barrett's oesophagus and that dietary interventions can also improve tissue repair, reduce inflammation, and improve general health.

Studies have shown that nutritional therapy is important when it comes to the health of the oesophagus. For example, dietary antioxidants like vitamin C and beta-carotene may prevent esophageal damage and lower the likelihood of Barrett's oesophagus progression, according to a comprehensive study published in the Journal of Gastroenterology and Hepatology. Furthermore, patients who have included nutritional therapy in their treatment plan attest to improvements in their overall quality of life, digestion, and reflux problems.

When incorporated into regular eating habits, nutritional therapy can provide real advantages for those with Barrett's oesophagus. Useful applications include meal planning where whole, unprocessed foods—such as fruits, vegetables, whole grains, and lean proteins—are given priority. Additionally, include anti-inflammatory foods like ginger and turmeric in meals can offer specific support for the health of the oesophagus.

Moving on to the study of herbal medicine, the application of botanical treatments provides an adjunctive method to traditional therapy, utilising the capacity of plant-derived components to promote esophageal health and general wellness.

Herbal Remedies and Their Efficacy

When it comes to the overall care of Barrett's oesophagus, investigating herbal therapies is especially important. For decades, herbal therapy has been a part of many traditional treatment systems. Lately, its potential benefits for the comprehensive care of Barrett's oesophagus are drawing more and more attention. Using reliable data to clarify their modes of action, evidence-based support, and useful applications, this section seeks to explore the effectiveness of herbal therapies in easing and supporting Barrett's oesophagus symptoms.

The main assertion being investigated is the possible effectiveness of herbal treatments in providing support and alleviation for the symptoms of Barrett's oesophagus. More specifically, this includes the use of herbal remedies to promote the integrity of the oesophagus tissue, reduce inflammation, and lessen reflux symptoms.

A wide range of plants and their extracts are used in herbal medicine; these extracts each contain distinct bioactive components that have been investigated for possible therapeutic effects on gastrointestinal health. A number of herbal therapies that are relevant to Barrett's oesophagus have drawn attention due to their antioxidant, anti-inflammatory, and mucosal-protective qualities. Notably, studies have looked into the use of herbs including marshmallow root, licorice, and slippery elm to ease esophageal irritation, lower inflammation, and promote mucosal healing. In addition, herbs like peppermint, ginger, and chamomile are known to assist the digestive system and lessen symptoms of reflux.

Numerous scientific studies that emphasise the bioactive ingredients and mechanisms of action of herbal treatments support their effectiveness in managing Barrett's oesophagus. For example, it has been demonstrated that slippery elm, a mucilaginous herb that is calming and anti-inflammatory, forms a protective layer over the lining of the oesophagus. Similarly, the anti-inflammatory and mucosal-protective qualities of licorice root, which contains flavonoids and glycyrrhizin, may help people with Barrett's oesophagus. Further research has examined the possibility of the volatile oils in peppermint and chamomile to relax the esophageal sphincter and reduce reflux symptoms, which could help with overall symptom reduction.

Although there are clear advantages to using herbal medicines to control Barrett's oesophagus, it's crucial to be aware of any potential drawbacks and contraindications before using them. Herbal remedies have the potential to worsen underlying medical issues or interfere with prescription drugs. Moreover, the efficacy and safety of herbal products may be impacted by variations in their quality and standardisation, which calls for careful assessment.

In order to allay worries about the effectiveness and safety of herbal remedies, it is critical to stress the need of seeking advice from licenced healthcare providers, especially naturopathic doctors or integrative medicine practitioners, before incorporating herbal preparations into the treatment of Barrett's oesophagus. Moreover, stringent quality control procedures and evidence-based recommendations can guarantee the dependability and safety of herbal products, minimising hazards and optimising their therapeutic potential.

Apart from the herbal therapies listed before, an increasing amount of preclinical and clinical research indicates that other botanicals including fenugreek, aloe vera, and turmeric may also be able to alleviate the symptoms of Barrett's oesophagus. The potential usefulness of these herbal medicines in promoting esophageal health is attributed to their varied modes of action, which include anti-inflammatory, antioxidant, and gastroprotective properties.

To sum up, investigating herbal treatments for Barrett's oesophagus management reveals a range of promising treatment alternatives that may help with symptom relief and maintain the health of the oesophagus. Although the many bioactive components included in herbal preparations provide pathways for tissue support and symptom treatment, integration of these compounds into comprehensive management strategies requires caution and well-informed decision-making. Herbal medicines can become useful supplements to traditional treatment through thorough evaluation based on evidence and well-informed advice, enhancing the comprehensive care of patients with Barrett's oesophagus.

Healing Through Yoga and Movement

The main goal of this section is to clarify how people with Barrett's oesophagus can benefit greatly from the integration of yoga and movement practises, giving them a comprehensive approach to controlling their illness. In addition to addressing the particular difficulties connected with Barrett's oesophagus, this section attempts to provide readers with useful skills for improving their physical, mental, and emotional well-being by detailing certain yoga asanas, breathing exercises, and mindful movement practises.

People with Barrett's oesophagus should be aware of their physical capabilities and any restrictions or contraindications imposed by their condition in order to participate in the suggested yoga and movement routines. To further enhance a secure and favourable practise environment, loose-fitting apparel, a supportive and comfy yoga mat, and a calm, well-ventilated area are advised.

For Barrett's oesophagus care, yoga and movement practises are integrated in a multifaceted way that addresses physical discomfort, stress reduction, and overall well-being. The method combines focused breathing techniques, mild yoga poses, and modest motions designed to improve esophageal health and reduce discomfort. This section lays the groundwork for an all-encompassing and empowering self-care regimen by summarising the essential elements and advantages of yoga and movement for people with Barrett's oesophagus.

* : Soft yoga poses that improve digestion, release tension in the upper body, and encourage relaxation include supported inversions, seated twists, and gentle backbends. These poses are especially chosen to provide mild support for people with Barrett's oesophagus, preventing undue pressure on the abdomen and oesophagus.

* : Using mindful breathing methods, such diaphragmatic and alternate nostril breathing, can improve respiration, lower stress levels, and induce calmness. Through the development of respiratory

efficiency and breath awareness, these strategies hope to promote a state of harmonious body-mind balance.

* : Incorporating subtle movement techniques can help with circulation, reduce muscle tension, and increase body awareness. Examples of these techniques include mindful walking, somatic motions, and gentle stretching. Because of the accessibility and adaptability of these motions, people with Barrett's oesophagus can participate in physical activity that improves their general well-being without making their symptoms worse.

- : When doing yoga and other movement practises, people with Barrett's oesophagus must respect their physical limits and cultivate self-compassion. It's important to avoid strong or vigorous motions that could make discomfort worse, and adjustments should be made to meet the needs of each individual.

- : People with Barrett's oesophagus are recommended to speak with their healthcare practitioners before beginning any new physical practises, especially if they already have any musculoskeletal or respiratory issues. This proactive approach guarantees that the practises selected are in line with their general well-being and medical considerations.

- : When doing yoga and other movement activities, people should be cognizant of any pain or symptoms they may be experiencing. To avoid aggravating reflux symptoms, adjustments or substitute techniques should be taken into consideration if specific postures or movements cause discomfort.

Self-assessment of symptom reduction, improved stress management, and overall well-being can validate the efficacy of yoga and movement activities in managing Barrett's oesophagus. As they adopt these techniques into their routine, people can keep track of their experiences and progress, noting any changes in symptom severity, emotional resilience, and physical comfort.

In conclusion, a comprehensive and powerful approach to self-care is provided to people with Barrett's oesophagus by the combination of yoga and movement practises. Gentle yoga asanas, mindful breathing exercises, and subtle movement practises can help people develop a stronger sense of well-being, improve their physical resilience, and create a body-mind harmony. The ability to practise yoga and movement mindfully, with self-compassion and with knowledgeable direction, can be a valuable addition to the overall management of Barrett's oesophagus.

Mental Health and Emotional Well-being

Coping With Chronic Illness

It's critical to address the mental and emotional burdens that frequently accompany a diagnosis of Barrett's oesophagus as people deal with the intricacies and difficulties of managing a chronic condition. Handling the day-to-day effects of a chronic illness such as Barrett's oesophagus requires a multimodal strategy that includes comprehending the background, characterising the issue, emphasising possible outcomes, presenting workable solutions, outlining strategies for implementation, exhibiting previous or anticipated results, and optionally debating alternate solutions.

Barrett's Esophagus is a disorder that causes alterations to the esophageal lining and presents major obstacles to persons in their daily lives. Patients and their loved ones bear a great deal of suffering when the illness is linked to gastroesophageal reflux disease (GERD) and has the potential to proceed to esophageal cancer. Managing Barrett's oesophagus can have a significant psychological and emotional toll and calls for careful thought and useful intervention.

The main challenge that people with Barrett's oesophagus encounter is maintaining ongoing awareness and control over their illness. Anxiety, depression, and a general decline in life quality are possible manifestations of this. The psychological strain that patients endure is further compounded by the ambiguity surrounding the possible development of Barrett's oesophagus to cancer.

If people with Barrett's oesophagus do not receive treatment for the mental and emotional difficulties it presents, their general health may suffer. Increased stress and worry, social isolation, a diminished capacity to manage the physical symptoms of the illness, and perhaps non-adherence to dietary and lifestyle guidelines are a few examples of this.

Barrett's oesophagus presents mental and emotional difficulties that must be addressed with a comprehensive strategy that incorporates lifestyle changes, psychological assistance, and self-care techniques. Psychosocial therapies have shown potential in reducing the emotional discomfort that people with chronic illnesses endure. These interventions include support groups, mindfulness-based stress reduction, and cognitive-behavioral therapy.

Providing psychological support to people with Barrett's oesophagus requires cooperation between medical staff, mental health specialists, and the patients under treatment. Referrals for patients seeking specialised support for managing chronic illnesses might be made to psychologists or counsellors who can provide individualised care. Additionally, in order to recognise and handle any new psychological issues, healthcare professionals might include routine mental health evaluations into the overall care plan.

Research has indicated that including psychological support into the treatment of people with long-term illnesses can result in better mental health, less anxiety and sadness, and better compliance with prescribed treatment plans. Barrett's esophageal reflux patients may benefit from improved coping strategies, a more optimistic outlook, and an improved quality of life by treating the mental and emotional aspects of the disease.

While psychological assistance is essential for managing the mental and emotional difficulties associated with Barrett's oesophagus, complementary therapies like music therapy, art therapy, or relaxation techniques may also be helpful. These methods can supplement conventional psychological treatments and provide people other ways to take control of their emotional health.

In summary, managing the psychological and emotional difficulties associated with having Barrett's oesophagus requires a comprehensive strategy that recognises the significant influence the illness has on people's mental health. People with Barrett's oesophagus can create a resilient mindset that supports their general well-being and better negotiate the intricacies of their illness by incorporating psychological support, encouraging self-care practises, and creating a collaborative healthcare environment.

Support Systems and Communities

People who are managing Barrett's oesophagus frequently struggle with the psychological and emotional effects of having a chronic illness. This diagnosis has implications for mental health, emotional stability, and social interactions in addition to the disease's outward symptoms. Therefore, it becomes imperative to investigate the importance of locating and engaging with communities and support networks that can provide emotional support, guidance, and a pool of common experiences for those navigating the intricacies of Barrett's oesophagus.

Living with Barrett's oesophagus involves more than just the physical components of the illness; it also significantly affects people's emotional and psychological health. The realisation of the complex nature of living with a chronic illness leads to the need to address the emotional burden and look for groups and support structures. Emotional support is becoming a crucial component of patients' holistic care as they work to manage their disease.

The main problem that people who have Barrett's oesophagus face is that because their illness is persistent, they may feel alone and distressed. Elevated anxiety, despair, and alienation might result from the worry of the disease progressing, the difficulty of controlling symptoms, and the impact on day-to-day life. People who have Barrett's oesophagus may find their overall quality of life greatly reduced by these emotional difficulties.

Untreated emotional distress related to Barrett's oesophagus can lead to a variety of negative outcomes for sufferers, such as declining mental well-being, diminished ability to withstand the condition's hardships, damaged relationships with others, and possibly even treatment plan non-compliance. In addition, the lack of a network of support can worsen people's emotional suffering, which exacerbates the detrimental effects on their wellbeing.

Getting involved in communities and support networks presents a viable strategy for addressing the psychological and emotional difficulties related to Barrett's oesophagus. People who connect with others who have gone through similar things as they can provide them with reassurance, understanding, and useful guidance that can improve their emotional health. Communities and support networks can offer a feeling of acceptance and understanding, which is crucial in preventing the emotional isolation that people with long-term illnesses frequently endure.

The establishment of support networks and community involvement entails a number of tactics meant to provide pathways for people living with Barrett's oesophagus to interact with others. This can involve being a part of online forums, attending educational events that encourage communication and information sharing, or joining support groups designed especially for people with Barrett's oesophagus. Healthcare professionals are essential in pointing people in the direction of these support networks and highlighting their importance in fostering emotional health.

Studies and firsthand accounts have demonstrated that involvement in communities and support networks can benefit those with long-term illnesses. Better coping strategies, less feelings of loneliness, more emotional resilience, and a stronger sense of empowerment in controlling their illness are a few possible results. Moreover, people who interact with support networks frequently report being more inclined to follow treatment regimens and adopt healthy lifestyle choices.

While communities and support networks provide priceless emotional support, other options include participating in creative treatments, like music or art therapy, to supplement the emotional nutrition provided by support networks. Developing a strong social support network, practising mindfulness, and engaging in self-care activities can all help strengthen the emotional resilience of people with Barrett's oesophagus.

It is impossible to overestimate the importance of helping people with Barrett's oesophagus identify and engage with support networks and communities. People can gain access to a plethora of shared experiences, helpful counsel, and emotional support by actively participating in these networks, all of which enhance general well-being. A caring community can be a ray of hope and courage for people navigating the challenges of caring for Barrett's oesophagus, encouraging empathy and solidarity in the face of hardship.

To sum up, the psychological and emotional difficulties associated with having Barrett's oesophagus require the development of communities and support networks that provide understanding, a wealth of experiences, and useful guidance. People can find comfort, empowerment, and emotional support by embracing the collective strength of these networks, which will ultimately lead to a more robust and richer journey of managing their disease.

Therapy and Counseling Approaches

Chronic illnesses like Barrett's oesophagus require more than just medical therapies and physical therapy to be managed. It includes an all-encompassing strategy that recognises the complex interactions that exist between the body, mind, and emotions. We will look at a variety of treatment and counselling philosophies in this part that provide people with Barrett's oesophagus with much-needed assistance and direction. By addressing the psychological and emotional aspects of the illness, these methods seek to give people the skills they need to improve their resilience and general well-being.

Family therapy, supportive counselling, mindfulness-based therapies, cognitive-behavioral therapy (CBT), and other therapeutic modalities are used in the management of Barrett's oesophagus. In order to support people with chronic diseases' emotional well-being, resilience, and adaptive coping mechanisms, each of these modalities has a unique but connected function.

a. Cognitive Behavioral Therapy (CBT) is a well-known treatment modality that aims to detect and alter dysfunctional thought patterns and behaviours. CBT can be very helpful for people with Barrett's oesophagus in treating their anxiety, despair, and negative thought patterns related to the illness. By focusing on behavioural patterns and cognitive distortions, cognitive behavioural therapy (CBT) gives people useful tools to deal with the emotional fallout from their diagnosis and deal with the difficulties of having a chronic condition.

b. The foundation of CBT is the idea that our feelings, thoughts, and actions are all interrelated. When Barrett's oesophagus is present, people may feel more anxious about the possibility that the illness will worsen, about experiencing symptoms, or about their long-term health. Through cognitive behavioural therapy (CBT), people can learn to recognise and question these unsettling ideas, swapping them out for more logical and helpful viewpoints. Furthermore, CBT methods like stress management and relaxation training give people practical tools to reduce emotional distress and improve their general well-being.

c. Several studies have shown that cognitive behavioural therapy (CBT) is effective in treating anxiety and depression in the setting of long-term medical problems. Studies carried out on patients suffering from gastrointestinal problems, such as Barrett's oesophagus, have demonstrated that cognitive behavioural therapy (CBT) interventions result in noteworthy decreases in anxiety levels, greater coping mechanisms, and improved quality of life. In addition, testimonies from those who have received CBT demonstrate its revolutionary influence on their emotional fortitude and capacity to manage the mental obstacles linked to long-term medical conditions.

d. CBT has real-world uses for people with Barrett's oesophagus outside of the therapeutic context. Through cognitive behavioural therapy (CBT), people can learn effective stress management techniques, build adaptive coping strategies, and enhance their emotional regulation. These newly acquired skills enable people to face their emotional difficulties head-on and provide them the means to participate in self-care activities that advance their general wellbeing. People can proactively address the emotional effect of their disease and cultivate a sense of empowerment in controlling their health by incorporating cognitive behavioural therapy (CBT) principles into their daily life.

After discussing CBT, we move on to the next therapy strategy that may be useful in helping people with Barrett's oesophagus: mindfulness-based therapies.

a. A variety of techniques that focus on developing acceptance, nonjudgmental attention, and present-moment awareness are included in mindfulness-based interventions. These therapies, which include mindful breathing exercises, yoga, and mindfulness meditation, give people with Barrett's oesophagus the chance to become more emotionally resilient and self-aware in the face of the difficulties associated with their illness.

b. Within the framework of Barrett's Esophagus, mindfulness-based therapies offer people a transforming framework to manage the uncertainties that come with their health journey and to navigate their emotional experiences. Adopting mindfulness techniques helps people become more emotionally balanced and accepting by teaching them to notice their thoughts and feelings without getting caught up in them. Additionally, mindfulness practises can assist people in reducing the stress brought on by doctor's appointments, treatment plans, and the impact of their illness on day-to-day living.

c. Studies on the use of mindfulness-based therapies in the treatment of chronic illnesses have shown how effective they are at lowering psychological discomfort, boosting emotional health, and strengthening coping mechanisms. Research conducted on patients with gastrointestinal disorders has demonstrated the beneficial effects of mindfulness techniques on anxiety reduction, emotional resilience building, and psychological well-being. Testimonials from people who have included mindfulness into their daily routines highlight the way in which it fosters a more self-aware and compassionate attitude to handling the emotional difficulties associated with chronic illness.

d. Mindfulness-based therapies have real-world uses outside of scheduled practise sessions. People who have Barrett's oesophagus can incorporate mindfulness practises into their daily lives by practising mindful breathing in times of high anxiety or doing gentle yoga to release physical tension. People can develop increased emotional resilience, self-compassion, and adaptive coping skills by practising mindfulness, which will enable them to deal with the emotional intricacies of their condition more calmly and easily.

After discussing mindfulness-based interventions in detail, we go on to the next therapeutic approach, which is supportive therapy.

A. Supportive counselling provides a secure and understanding environment for people with Barrett's oesophagus to communicate their feelings, worries, and challenges associated with their illness. The goals of this therapeutic technique are to provide emotional support, validate the experiences of individuals, and cultivate acceptance and understanding.

b. When it comes to Barrett's oesophagus, supportive counselling gives patients a way to work with the emotional effects of their diagnosis, course of treatment, and any unknowns surrounding their illness. Individuals can learn coping mechanisms, explore their emotional experiences, and get validation for their struggles by forming a therapeutic alliance with a caring counsellor. Furthermore, supportive counselling can help people reframe how they see their situation, which can help them feel resilient and hopeful in the midst of hardship.

c. Studies on the effectiveness of supportive counselling in managing chronic illnesses have highlighted the ways in which it might lessen psychological discomfort, improve quality of life, and reduce emotional anguish. Research done on people with gastrointestinal disorders has shown how beneficial supportive counselling is for building emotional resilience, lowering feelings of loneliness, and encouraging adaptable coping mechanisms. Testimonials from clients who have received supportive counselling highlight the therapeutic approach's transformative power for improving the client's emotional well-being and capacity to deal with the difficulties of managing a chronic illness.

d. The cooperative interaction between clients and their counsellors is one of the practical uses of supportive therapy. People can explore their emotional experiences, create unique coping mechanisms, and strengthen their emotional resilience through supportive counselling. Additionally, as people navigate the emotional complexities of their health journey, the insights gained from supportive counselling sessions can empower people to integrate self-care practises, cultivate adaptive coping mechanisms, and foster a more compassionate and understanding relationship with themselves.

After discussing supportive counselling, we go on to the last type of therapy: family therapy.

a. Family therapy acknowledges the interdependence of family relationships and how they affect the emotional health of those who have Barrett's oesophagus. With the use of this treatment technique, family members can actively participate in helping the person managing the chronic condition with their emotional needs and support.

b. Family therapy provides a platform for people with Barrett's oesophagus and their families to manage the emotional effects of the diagnosis, the course of treatment, and the necessary lifestyle adaptations. Through family therapy, people can address issues related to communication, emotional support requirements, and how the condition affects family dynamics. Furthermore, family therapy offers a setting for the development of comprehension, compassion, and cooperative techniques for managing the emotional intricacies linked to long-term medical conditions.

c. Studies examining the effectiveness of family therapy in managing chronic illnesses have shown its capacity to ameliorate emotional support, augment communication within the family, and cultivate a heightened sense of comprehension and unity. Research involving people with gastrointestinal disorders has demonstrated the beneficial effects of family therapy in lowering stress within the family, enhancing coping mechanisms, and creating a nurturing atmosphere for the person with the long-term illness. Testimonials from patients and their families highlight how family therapy may be a game-changer in building resilience, strengthening family ties, and encouraging a more unified strategy for coping with the psychological effects of long-term illness.

d. The joint efforts of individuals and their families in resolving the emotional effect of Barrett's oesophagus are one of the practical applications of family therapy. Individuals and their families can improve understanding and cohesion, create emotional support, and learn effective communication techniques through family therapy. Family therapy furthermore offers a means of navigating the emotional intricacies of the disease as a cohesive unit, cultivating adaptable coping methods, empathy, and resilience that are advantageous to the individual as well as their support system of family members.

After delving into the specifics of every therapy and counselling modality, we have looked at the many approaches that could be helpful in helping people with Barrett's oesophagus. These methods, which range from family therapy and supportive counselling to mindfulness-based therapies and cognitive-behavioral therapy, all add up to a thorough framework for addressing the psychological and emotional aspects of having a chronic health condition. Through the integration of these therapy modalities into their comprehensive care, patients can develop adaptive coping mechanisms, emotional resilience, and an enhanced feeling of wellbeing while navigating the challenges associated with managing Barrett's oesophagus.

Finally, the investigation of treatment and counselling modalities for people with Barrett's oesophagus highlights the

Mind-Body Connection and Healing

In the field of healthcare and managing chronic illnesses, there has been a growing interest in and investigation of the mind-body link and its role in healing. In the context of Barrett's Esophagus, comprehending the complex interactions between mental and physical health has important ramifications for people managing the intricacies of their illness. In order to better understand the significant impact that mental health has on Barrett's oesophagus care, this chapter will look at the ways in which psychological factors can affect symptoms, treatment results, and general quality of life. Through clarifying the relationship between the body and mind within the framework of Barrett's oesophagus, this investigation seeks to give people useful knowledge and techniques to improve their resilience and overall well-being.

This chapter will investigate the main hypothesis, which is that Barrett's oesophagus requires comprehensive therapy that heavily relies on the mind-body connection. In particular, the psychological aspects of the illness can have a substantial impact on symptom experiences, adherence to therapy, and general health outcomes; for this reason, a comprehensive strategy that incorporates mental health into the care paradigm is required.

Examining the impact of psychological variables on Barrett's oesophagus experience requires a review of empirical data and clinical observations. Studies have repeatedly shown how psychological health affects the symptomatology of gastrointestinal disorders, such as Barrett's oesophagus. Research has demonstrated, for example, that people who are more stressed and anxious may also have worsened symptoms like heartburn and regurgitation, indicating the complex relationship between mental and physical states. Moreover, the impact of psychological variables on treatment compliance and involvement with healthcare treatments highlights the extensive consequences of mental health in the handling of long-term illnesses.

Psychological health and the Barrett's esophageal experience are linked not just to symptomatology but also to treatment results and general quality of life. People who deal with chronic illnesses frequently deal with a wide range of emotional difficulties, such as worry about their future health, fear of symptoms, and anxiety over the course of the disease. The course of their illness can be greatly influenced by these emotional events in terms of treatment compliance, lifestyle changes, and interaction with medical professionals. Furthermore, the psychological effects of a chronic illness can penetrate many areas of a person's life, impacting their sense of general well-being, productivity at work, and interpersonal connections.

Although psychological health has a significant impact on Barrett's oesophagus care, it is important to recognise that every person's experience and reaction to the illness are unique. Certain individuals may exhibit exceptional resilience and adaptive coping techniques, thereby effectively reducing the influence of psychological factors on their treatment outcomes and symptom experiences. Furthermore, because of the intricate relationship between the mind and body, it is imperative to recognise that managing chronic illnesses is a complex process, involving the intersection of biological, environmental, and social factors with psychological well-being to influence an individual's overall health trajectory.

Although individual responses vary, the overall evidence highlights the significant impact of the mind-body connection on Barrett's oesophagus care. By acknowledging and addressing the psychological aspects of the illness, people might be better equipped to manage their health, interact with treatment options more skillfully, and maintain their sense of wellbeing in the face of obstacles brought on by their diagnosis.

Apart from empirical studies, the personal accounts and testimonials of individuals who have Barrett's Esophagus provide significant insights into the significant influence of psychological health on their ability to manage their condition. Personal narratives frequently highlight how important coping mechanisms, emotional fortitude, and supportive networks were in influencing the way that individuals experienced life with a chronic illness. In the context of Barrett's Esophagus, these stories serve as moving reminders of the complex interactions that occur between the mind and body.

The analysis of the mind-body relationship in relation to Barrett's oesophagus concludes by highlighting the critical role that psychological health plays in symptom experiences, treatment results, and general quality of life. People can develop adaptive coping mechanisms, interact with their healthcare journey more effectively, and create a stronger sense of well-being despite the challenges of managing a chronic health condition by recognising and addressing the psychological aspects of the condition. This highlights the critical role that an integrated, holistic approach—which includes mental health—plays in providing comprehensive Barrett's oesophagus management.

Overcoming Anxiety and Depression

Beyond their outward symptoms, chronic diseases may pose a variety of other difficulties. Among these difficulties, anxiety and depression together can have a serious negative effect on a person's general health and quality of life. Understanding the complex interactions that exist between mental health and chronic illness is essential, especially when it comes to treating diseases like Barrett's oesophagus. This chapter delves into the intricacies of sadness and anxiety in the setting of long-term illness, examining any possible ramifications and offering practical management techniques. Through clarifying the significant impact of mental health on the treatment of chronic illnesses, this investigation seeks to enable people to travel the path of health with greater resilience and improved health.

Psychological problems such as anxiety and sadness are common and often coexist with chronic illnesses like Barrett's oesophagus. These mental health problems can arise or worsen as a result of the stress of managing a chronic illness, which presents major challenges to people who are trying to keep their physical and mental health in check. In addition to increasing people's emotional suffering, the co-existence of anxiety and depression creates obstacles to good disease management, treatment compliance, and general health outcomes.

Untreated anxiety and depression have a variety of negative effects on managing chronic illnesses. These mental health issues may be linked to increased stress, worsening physical problems, and a lower standard of living. In addition, people who struggle with anxiety and depression may find it difficult to follow treatment plans, communicate with medical professionals, and successfully make lifestyle changes, which could hinder their overall health trajectory.

Sustaining anxiety and sadness in the face of chronic illness requires a multimodal strategy that incorporates psychological health into the paradigm of treatment. It is imperative to employly evidence-based ways to tackle mental health issues in order to bolster individuals' resilience and augment their ability to adeptly manage the intricacies of their health journey.

When it comes to managing chronic diseases, a range of interventions are used to address anxiety and depression. These include pharmaceutical treatments, lifestyle adjustments, and psychological therapy. Furthermore, self-care techniques and the development of a compassionate and encouraging healthcare environment can be extremely important in enabling people to effectively address and manage their mental health issues.

Implementing treatments targeted at managing anxiety and depression in the setting of chronic illness can provide favourable results, as research and clinical data regularly show. People who participate in complete, integrated treatments that include mental health strategies have been shown to have gains in general quality of life, improved adherence to treatment, and reduced intensity of symptoms.

While medication and psychological counselling are frequently used to treat anxiety and depression, other strategies including exercise programmes, mindfulness-based interventions, and complementary therapies provide people with more ways to effectively manage their mental health issues. Assessing the appropriateness and effectiveness of various substitute approaches can offer people a wide range of choices for managing their chronic illness while attending to their psychological well-being.

To sum up, managing anxiety and depression in the context of chronic illness is a complicated but important part of general health and wellbeing. In the midst of the difficulties of managing a chronic illness, people can improve their resilience, lessen the effects of psychological difficulties, and foster a stronger sense of well-being by acknowledging the significant impact that mental health has on disease management and putting evidence-based strategies into practise. This emphasises how important it is to manage chronic diseases holistically and integratedly, taking mental health into account.

Self-Help Techniques for Emotional Regulation

This section aims to provide self-help methods for stress management and emotional control. The goal is to lead the reader through each stage of the process by offering a step-by-step blueprint of activities and procedures in order to accomplish a particular goal: the capacity to successfully control emotions and handle stress by using self-help techniques.

Prior to exploring the particular methods of emotional regulation, people should be open to practising self-awareness and self-reflection. A quiet place for reflection and a notebook or journal for jotting down ideas and feelings can also be helpful. Success in stress management and emotional regulation also requires an open mind and a dedication to putting the recommended approaches into practise.

Realizing how thoughts, emotions, and behaviours are interconnected is the first step towards using self-help approaches to manage stress and regulate emotions. This comprehensive outline will give a quick summary of the processes in the process, which include cognitive restructuring, mindfulness exercises, and relaxation methods.

1. : Cultivating mindfulness, or the discipline of being present and aware of one's thoughts and feelings without passing judgement, is the cornerstone of emotional control. Methods like body scanning, mindfulness meditation, and deep breathing can help people become more emotionally aware and learn how to deal with their emotions in a composed and controlled way.

2. : This level entails recognising and combating harmful thought patterns that fuel emotional suffering. People can reframe their perceptions and ease emotional upheaval by investigating the veracity of negative beliefs and replace them with well-balanced, sensible thoughts.

3. : Relaxation techniques including progressive muscle relaxation, yoga, and visualisation can be useful tools for lowering stress and fostering emotional balance. By addressing the physiological signs of stress and anxiety, these methods seek to promote serenity and calmness.

4. : An essential component of emotional control is promoting acceptance of one's emotions and self-compassion. Reducing the impact of stressful emotions and promoting emotional resilience can be achieved by accepting emotions without passing judgement on them and by showing love and understanding to oneself.

- Consistency is key: It takes consistent practise of these methods to become proficient in emotional management.

- Patience and persistence: Learning how to control your emotions is a skill that takes time and practise. It is crucial that people have self-compassion while they work through this process.

- Seek professional guidance if needed: Self-help methods can be helpful, but people who are experiencing serious emotional distress or mental health issues should get help from licenced mental health experts.

A discernible decrease in the frequency and intensity of upsetting feelings, as well as an improved capacity to react calmly and clearly in difficult circumstances, serve as indicators that emotional regulation is working.

Practicing self-help approaches for emotional regulation can present a number of common difficulties, such as reluctance to change, scepticism about the techniques' efficacy, and trouble maintaining consistency. Reexamining the justification for practising emotional control, asking peers or mental health specialists for help, and modifying the methods to better meet personal preferences and requirements are some possible solutions to these problems.

To sum up, developing self-help skills for stress relief and emotional control is a life-changing experience that enables people to use their own inner resources for emotional health. Through the use of mindfulness, cognitive restructuring, relaxation techniques, and self-compassion, individuals can develop resilience, improve their emotional balance, and more skillfully negotiate the intricacies of their inner world.

Building Resilience and Positivity

This section's objective is to examine strategies for developing resilience and keeping a positive mindset in the face of health obstacles. The goal is to lead the reader through each stage and accomplish a certain goal by offering a step-by-step road map of actions and procedures: the capacity to develop resilience and optimism in the face of health-related challenges.

It is crucial that people begin this journey with an open mind and a readiness to adjust before diving into the specific tactics for sustaining happiness and building resilience. In addition, success in developing resilience and preserving positivity requires a supportive environment, access to tools that promote personal development, and a dedication to self-care.

Realizing the connection between physical and mental well-being is the first step in developing resilience and retaining optimism in the face of health issues. This general synopsis will give an overview of the processes in the process, which include developing a supportive network, changing one's perspective, and developing coping mechanisms.

1. : Reframing adversity as a chance for learning and progress is a key component of developing a resilient attitude. A positive outlook and the understanding that problems are only temporary roadblocks rather than insurmountable roadblocks can help people develop resilience and improve their capacity to face health-related challenges head-on and with grace and resolve.

2. : Creating useful coping mechanisms is essential to staying upbeat when facing health issues. Stress management and emotional well-being can be effectively enhanced by employing strategies including practising gratitude, rephrasing unfavourable ideas, and partaking in joyful and fulfilling activities.

3. : Making self-care a priority is crucial for preserving optimism and developing resilience. Resilience can be strengthened and a positive outlook can be fostered in the face of health-related challenges by partaking in activities that nourish the body, mind, and spirit, such as exercise, a balanced diet, enough sleep, and relaxation.

4. : Creating and maintaining a network of family, friends, and medical professionals who are supportive can be extremely helpful in times of need by offering emotional support and encouragement. Making connections with people who can relate to and validate one's experiences can help one feel resilient and like they belong when facing health-related obstacles.

- Embrace the power of perspective: Understand that deliberate changes in viewpoint and attitude toward adversity are necessary to promote resilience and positivity.

- Practice self-compassion: Treat yourself with compassion and recognise the fortitude and tenacity required to overcome obstacles related to your health.

- Seek professional support if needed: Although one can create personal resilience and positivity, consulting healthcare professionals can offer further tools and assistance.

An improved capacity to adjust to health-related setbacks, an increased ability to find joy and purpose despite difficulties, and a sense of empowerment in negotiating the intricacies of health management with resilience and optimism are all indicators of successful resilience and positivity.

Those who are trying to develop resilience and keep a positive outlook in the face of health difficulties frequently struggle with emotions of overwhelm, self-doubt, and loneliness. In order to overcome these obstacles, one may need to exercise self-compassion, look for peer support, and seek professional assistance while navigating difficult feelings and situations.

In summary, developing resilience and optimism in the face of health difficulties is a life-changing process that enables people to manage their health with grace, courage, and tenacity. People can develop resilience and keep a positive attitude in the face of health-related challenges by adopting mindset adjustments, practical coping mechanisms, self-care routines, and building a supportive network.

Lifestyle Modifications and Home Remedies

Creating a Barrett's-Friendly Home

This chapter's goal is to assist those who have Barrett's oesophagus in setting up their homes in a way that facilitates the management of their illness. Readers will be able to improve their lifestyle and reduce potential triggers by strategically altering their living environment, thereby promoting general well-being.

Prior to starting the process of making a house that is Barrett's-friendly, it is critical to evaluate the existing living space and pinpoint any possible areas for enhancement. Changing the kitchen, dining room, bedroom, and general household routines may be necessary for this. Furthermore, it's critical to have a fundamental grasp of the illness and how to treat it, including dietary guidelines, lifestyle adjustments, and the significance of stress reduction.

Making a house Barrett's friendly requires a thorough strategy that takes into account many facets of daily life. This include making the kitchen as Barrett's-friendly as possible, establishing a calm and comfortable sleeping space, putting stress-reduction techniques into action, and making sure the entire living area is suitable for efficiently managing the illness.

1. Optimizing the Kitchen for Barrett's-Friendly Meals:

- Clearing out Trigger Foods: Start by determining which foods in the pantry and refrigerator are triggers, such as spicy, acidic, and fatty foods, and remove them.

- Stocking Up on Barrett's-Friendly Foods: In order to promote a healthy and balanced diet, introduce Barrett's-friendly foods such lean proteins, whole grains, fruits, and vegetables.

- Investing in Meal Preparation Tools: To make Barrett's-friendly meal preparation easier, think about spending money on appliances like a food steamer, a smoothie mixer, and portion control tools.

2. Creating a Soothing and Restful Bedroom Environment:

- Minimizing Light and Noise: To create a calm sleep environment, use blackout curtains and use white noise machines or earplugs.

- Choosing the Right Bedding: Choose pillows and bedding that are hypoallergenic to reduce the possibility of objects causing acid reflux while you sleep.

- Implementing Relaxation Techniques: Before going to bed, use relaxation techniques like deep breathing exercises, meditation, and light stretching to help you unwind and get a good night's sleep.

3. Implementing Stress-Reducing Practices:

- Designating Relaxation Areas: To promote stress reduction, establish specific spaces for relaxation in your house, such as a comfortable reading nook or a meditation place.

- Incorporating Aromatherapy: Throughout the house, use diffusers and essential oils to create a relaxing atmosphere that encourages relaxation.

- Exploring Stress-Relieving Activities: To effectively control stress levels, encourage participation in stress-relieving activities like yoga, tai chi, or walks in the outdoors.

4. Ensuring a Conducive Living Space:

- Decluttering and Organizing: Living areas can be made more organised and serene by decluttering, which can help people feel less stressed.

- Creating a Comfortable Dining Area: Create a welcoming and cosy dining space that encourages mindful eating and complements Barrett's-friendly cuisine.

- Before starting a new exercise programme or making big nutritional changes, it's crucial to speak with a medical practitioner or a qualified dietitian, especially for those who are managing Barrett's oesophagus.

- To guarantee that the meals are nutrient-balanced and in line with the demands of the individual, think about consulting a nutritionist when remodelling the kitchen for Barrett's-friendly dishes.

- It's best for people with Barrett's oesophagus to raise the head of the bed in order to avoid acid reflux as they sleep.

Those who successfully create a Barrett's-friendly environment can track their general health and symptoms over time. This could entail monitoring stress levels, food triggers, sleep patterns, and general home comfort.

Identifying trigger foods, keeping a stress-relieving atmosphere, and resisting lifestyle changes are common issues that can come up when making a house that is Barrett's friendly. In these situations, getting help from medical professionals, joining support groups, or consulting with professionals in stress management and home organising can all offer helpful advice and answers.

To sum up, designing a home that is Barrett's friendly is a complex procedure that includes maximising a number of areas of everyday life in order to facilitate Barrett's oesophagus management. Through deliberate attention to the kitchen, bedroom, stress reduction techniques, and general living area, people suffering from Barrett's oesophagus can improve their entire quality of life and well-being.

Effective Sleep Hygiene Practices

The maintenance of good sleep hygiene practises is essential for maintaining general wellbeing when controlling Barrett's oesophagus. Not only does getting enough sleep promote mental and physical renewal, but it also helps control Barrett's oesophagus symptoms. This extensive list of good sleep hygiene techniques is intended to provide people with useful tools to

a. The Impact of Consistent Sleep Patterns

b. Keeping a regular sleep pattern, which includes set wake-up and bedtimes, aids in the regulation of the circadian rhythm, the body's internal clock. Consistency in sleep promotes overall well-being and greater sleep quality by supporting the body's natural circadian rhythm. This internal rhythm can be upset by irregular sleep patterns, which can make it difficult to get to sleep and stay asleep through the night.

c. Consistent sleep schedules are beneficial for both overall health and higher sleep quality, as research studies have repeatedly shown. Testimonials from people who have kept up regular sleep schedules also highlight the beneficial effect on their capacity to successfully manage the symptoms of Barrett's oesophagus.

d. People can put this into practise by creating a sleep routine that works for them and sticking to it every day, including on the weekends. To tell the body it's time to get ready for sleep, this may entail establishing a wind-down routine and a set bedtime and wake-up time.

a. The Importance of Wind-Down Activities

b. Before going to bed, doing peaceful activities might help the body adjust from awake to sleep. This could be curling up with a book, having a warm bath, doing some light stretching, or practising some relaxation methods like progressive muscle relaxation or meditation. By lowering tension and anxiety, these activities help the body and mind get ready for a good night's sleep.

c. Research has indicated that implementing bedtime rituals can enhance both the onset and quality of sleep. Testimonials from Barrett's Oesophagus sufferers who have managed their illness better by integrating peaceful sleep rituals into their daily routines attest to the beneficial effects.

d. People can incorporate activities that encourage relaxation into a regular nightly pattern by identifying relaxing bedtime habits. The body can be signalled to relax and get ready for sleep by establishing a calm and regular pre-sleep habit.

a. Creating a Sleep-Conducive Environment

b. The setting of the bedroom is quite important for encouraging sound sleep. Variations in temperature, noise levels, and lighting can all have a big effect on how well you sleep. Making the bedroom as quiet, dark, and comfortably cool as possible will help ensure that you can sleep through the night. This can entail lowering noise levels, utilising blackout curtains, and regulating the temperature of the space to promote sleep.

c. High-quality sleep is facilitated by an ideal bedroom environment, as scientific research has demonstrated. Testimonials from people who are in charge of managing Barrett's oesophagus also highlight how having a bedroom that is suitable to sleep helps them manage their disease.

d. People can improve the atmosphere in their bedrooms by making small but effective adjustments, such changing the lighting, buying cosy cushions and bedding, and reducing noise. These adjustments can aid in establishing a calm and relaxing sleeping environment, which is beneficial for efficiently controlling the symptoms of Barrett's oesophagus.

a. The Influence of Stimulants on Sleep Quality

b. Caffeine, nicotine, and alcohol are examples of stimulants that might prevent the body from going into restorative sleep. Specifically, caffeine has a strong effect on sleep since it can stay in the body for several hours, interfering with the sleep-wake cycle. Reducing the amount of stimulants and other substances used, particularly before bed, might improve overall sleep hygiene and the quality of the sleep.

c. The disruption of sleep patterns caused by stimulants and drugs is a topic that is frequently addressed in scientific literature. The benefits of cutting back on stimulants in terms of improving sleep and controlling Barrett's oesophagus are also highlighted in the testimonies of those who manage the condition.

d. People can adopt doable tactics to restrict the amount of stimulants and substances they consume. Some of these tactics include limiting alcohol intake and staying away from items with caffeine and nicotine several hours before going to bed. These modifications can help with Barrett's oesophagus management and enhance the quality of your sleep.

a. The Role of Relaxation in Sleep Induction

b. Deep breathing exercises, progressive muscle relaxation, and guided imagery are a few examples of relaxation techniques that can help calm the body and mind and ease the transition into sleep. These methods encourage relaxation by easing tension and stress, which are frequent sleep-inducing factors. Relaxation techniques can help prime the body for sound sleep when incorporated into the nighttime routine.

c. The effectiveness of relaxation techniques in enhancing sleep onset and mitigating sleep disruptions has been shown by clinical trials. The benefits of relaxation techniques for improving sleep quality and coping with Barrett's oesophagus are further demonstrated by the testimonies of those who manage the condition.

d. People can include relaxation techniques into their evening routines by setting aside time for peaceful pursuits like progressive muscle relaxation or deep breathing exercises before to going to bed. By reducing stress and fostering calm, these techniques can aid in better sleep hygiene and the treatment of Barrett's oesophagus symptoms.

a. Cultivating Sleep-Inducing Habits

b. Better sleep quality can be promoted by adopting sleep-inducing behaviours like making a cosy sleeping environment, keeping a good sleeping posture, and avoiding stimulating activities just before bed. By supporting the body's innate sleep processes, these practises help people sleep in a regular, restorative manner.

c. Studies have demonstrated the benefits of integrating sleep-promoting practises into everyday schedules, resulting in better sleep and general health. Testimonials from patients with Barrett's oesophagus also emphasise the advantages of implementing sleep-inducing practises in the process of learning how to properly manage the condition.

d. People can develop sleep-inducing behaviours by using techniques including creating a cosy sleeping environment, maintaining proper posture when sleeping, and refraining from stimulating activities like using electronics just before bed. These routines can help control Barrett's oesophagus and improve the quality of your sleep.

Making a smooth transition from one good sleep hygiene practise to the next leads people through a whole process of raising the quality of their sleep. Through the incorporation of these tactics into everyday life, people can strengthen their capacity to effectively manage Barrett's Oesophagus, promoting a comprehensive approach to overall health and symptom management.

Home Remedies for Symptom Relief

As we proceed with our investigation into all-encompassing treatment approaches for Barrett's oesophagus, we must also explore the domain of home remedies that provide comfort and symptom relief. When used in conjunction with other medical treatments, home remedies can offer further assistance in reducing pain and enhancing general health. With the help of this comprehensive list of natural remedies, people can better control the symptoms of Barrett's oesophagus and promote a comprehensive approach to the condition's care.

a. The Therapeutic Properties of Ginger

b. Because of its well-known anti-inflammatory and calming qualities, ginger is a useful natural treatment for Barrett's oesophagus. Its active ingredients, which include shogaol and gingerol, have anti-inflammatory properties that may lessen discomfort and irritation in the gastrointestinal system. Furthermore, ginger helps relieve and improve overall comfort by reducing nausea, a frequent symptom of Barrett's oesophagus.

c. Ginger's anti-inflammatory and anti-nausea properties have been confirmed by scientific research, indicating that it may be used as a home treatment for Barrett's oesophagus patients. Testimonials from those who have used ginger infusions regularly have emphasised how beneficial they are for general well-being and symptom relief.

d. To make a calming and healing beverage, anyone can make their own ginger infusions by steeping fresh ginger slices in hot water. Before or in between meals, consuming a ginger infusion may assist maintain digestive health and alleviate discomfort, which can improve symptom management.

a. The Soothing Effects of Aloe Vera

b. Because of its well-known calming and anti-inflammatory qualities, aloe vera juice may be able to help those who suffer with Barrett's oesophagus. Aloe vera's mucilaginous properties may coat the oesophagus in a protective manner, so lessening irritation and pain. Aloe vera also contains substances like acemannan, which have healing and immune-modulating qualities and support the health of the gastrointestinal system as a whole.

c. Aloe vera's anti-inflammatory and mucoprotective properties have been demonstrated by research, suggesting that it could be used as a DIY treatment for people with Barrett's oesophagus. Testimonials from people who have included aloe vera juice in their daily routine highlight the calming effects and how it helps with symptom relief.

d. People can add aloe vera juice to their daily routine by taking a small amount before meals, which may help with discomfort and promote the health of the oesophagus. To guarantee the medicinal effects of aloe vera juice, it is crucial to choose pure, high-quality juice.

a. The Calming Influence of Chamomile

b. The chamomile flower is used to make chamomile tea, which has relaxing and anti-inflammatory qualities that may help people with Barrett's oesophagus. The anti-inflammatory properties of chamomile's bioactive components, such as luteolin and apigenin, may lessen oesophageal discomfort and increase comfort. Furthermore, chamomile's calming qualities might aid in reducing tension and anxiety, enhancing general wellbeing.

c. Research has demonstrated that chamomile has anti-inflammatory and anxiolytic properties, which lends credence to its use as a home treatment for Barrett's oesophagus. Testimonials from those who have made chamomile tea a regular part of their regimen highlight the tea's relaxing effects and advantages for managing symptoms.

d. People can add chamomile tea to their daily routine as a calming brew to sip on before bed or during uncomfortable times to help reduce symptoms and encourage relaxation.

a. The Mucilaginous Properties of Marshmallow Root

b. Due to its mucilaginous properties, marshmallow root may provide some alleviation for Barrett's oesophagus sufferers. Marshmallow root's mucilage coats the lining of the oesophagus, possibly easing discomfort and lowering inflammation. Additionally, marshmallow root's anti-inflammatory qualities can help lessen the discomfort brought on by Barrett's oesophagus.

c. Scientific literature has acknowledged marshmallow root's mucilaginous and anti-inflammatory properties, which supports marshmallow root's use as a home treatment for Barrett's oesophagus patients. Testimonials from people who have used marshmallow root in their regimen attest to its calming qualities and ability to reduce symptoms.

d. To perhaps take use of marshmallow root's mucilaginous and anti-inflammatory qualities, people can make marshmallow root infusions or take marshmallow root supplements. Before adding marshmallow root to a routine, it is vital to consult a healthcare provider, particularly if there are any underlying medical issues or drugs being taken at the same time.

a. The Gastroprotective Effects of Licorice Root

b. Glycyrrhizin and flavonoids, two substances found in licorice root, have anti-inflammatory and gastroprotective qualities that may help people with Barrett's oesophagus. These bioactive ingredients may aid in symptom management by easing discomfort and oesophageal irritation. Furthermore, licorice root may improve mucosal protection and reduce inflammatory reactions, which can benefit gastrointestinal health.

c. Studies have clarified the anti-inflammatory and gastroprotective properties of licorice root, giving it a scientific basis for use as a home treatment for Barrett's oesophagus patients. Accounts from patients who have used licorice root in their treatment plan highlight the herb's ability to reduce pain and promote oesophageal health.

d. People can take supplements or infusions made from licorice root, but they should be aware of the prescribed dosage and any contraindications. Before using licorice root in one's regimen, it is important to speak with a healthcare provider, especially if there are any co-occurring medical issues or drugs.

a. The Soothing Influence of Slippery Elm

b. Derived from the inner bark of the Ulmus rubra tree, slippery elm has mucilaginous and demulcent qualities that may provide some help for Barrett's oesophagus sufferers. Along the lining of the oesophagus, slippery elm's mucilage creates a protective layer that may lessen discomfort and increase comfort. Moreover, slippery elm may have anti-inflammatory properties that help relieve Barrett's esophageal discomfort.

c. The mucilaginous and anti-inflammatory properties of slippery elm have been highlighted in scientific literature, indicating that it may be used as a home treatment for Barrett's oesophagus patients. Testimonials from people who have included slippery elm in their regimen of care highlight the calming effect and possibility for symptom relief.

d. To take advantage of slippery elm's mucilaginous and anti-inflammatory qualities, people can make infusions or take supplements of the plant. Before adding slippery elm to one's regimen, it is best to consult a healthcare provider, particularly if there are any underlying medical issues or drugs being taken at the same time.

Shifting from one homemade cure to another in a smooth manner leads people through a thorough process of treating Barrett's oesophagus symptoms. Through the incorporation of these DIY treatments into their daily routine, people may be able to reduce pain and improve their general state of health, which promotes a more comprehensive approach to managing symptoms.

Smoking Cessation and Alcohol Moderation

In the field of managing oesophageal health, the relationship between alcohol intake, smoking, and the advancement of Barrett's oesophagus is a major concern. Knowing how alcohol and tobacco affect Barrett's oesophagus becomes crucial as patients travel through their journey with the illness. This section explores the importance of giving up smoking and reducing alcohol intake, highlighting the possible negative effects of ongoing usage and providing doable solutions for success.

It has been determined that persistent alcohol and tobacco use plays a negative role in the development and aggravation of Barrett's oesophagus. Smoking exposes the oesophagus to a wide range of harmful substances, such as carcinogens, which can alter cells and raise the possibility of oesophageal cancer. Similar to this, drinking too much alcohol can irritate the lining of the oesophagus, causing inflammation and increasing the risk of oesophageal problems. Comprehending the significance of these behaviours in relation to Barrett's Oesophagus is imperative for efficient handling and general welfare.

Inadequate attention to the smoking and alcohol intake issues may lead to worsening symptoms and a higher chance of the disease developing in those with Barrett's oesophagus. Persistent smoking has the ability to maintain oesophageal cellular abnormalities, which may worsen Barrett's oesophagus and increase the risk of developing cancer. Similarly, long-term alcohol misuse can exacerbate oesophageal irritation and inflammation, making treatment less effective and increasing discomfort.

The key to reducing the damaging effects of alcohol and smoking on Barrett's oesophagus is to cut back on alcohol intake and stop smoking. People can greatly lower their chance of developing new oesophageal injury and improve the efficacy of their management strategy by changing these practises. Making the decision to stop smoking and drink in moderation can be crucial in fostering the health and wellbeing of the oesophagus.

It takes a multifaceted strategy to implement measures for alcohol moderation and smoking cessation. People can look into evidence-based smoking cessation programmes like support groups, counselling, and nicotine replacement treatment. By addressing the psychological and physiological aspects of nicotine addiction, these techniques seek to support individuals in making the shift from smoking to a smoke-free lifestyle. Furthermore, establishing a caring atmosphere and enlisting the aid of medical experts can offer priceless direction during the quitting process. Setting explicit limits on alcohol consumption, recognising triggers, and looking for substitute coping methods are essential stages in the context of alcohol moderation. Taking part in stress-relieving activities and asking friends and family for support might strengthen the will to limit alcohol use.

The benefits of alcohol moderation and quitting smoking for those with Barrett's oesophagus have been repeatedly shown by research and clinical observations. According to studies, quitting smoking lowers oesophageal inflammation and lowers the chance that the disease will worsen. Similarly, increases in overall quality of life and oesophageal discomfort are reported by individuals who effectively decrease their alcohol usage. Following these recommendations should result in a significant improvement in the condition of the oesophagus and a decrease in the intensity of symptoms associated with Barrett's oesophagus.

While reducing alcohol intake and quitting smoking are the main ways to address the effects of these behaviours on Barrett's oesophagus, other techniques like behavioural therapy, mindfulness exercises, and peer support groups can also be helpful. When using holistic modalities that prioritise emotional and stress management, people embarking on a journey to quit smoking and drink in moderation can benefit from extra levels of support.

It is crucial to emphasise the need of quitting smoking and drinking in moderation when people manage Barrett's oesophagus. People can take proactive measures to protect their oesophagus and improve their general health by adopting these tactics. The management of Barrett's oesophagus may have a bright future with the use of evidence-based strategies and an unwavering commitment to reform..

Managing Weight for Optimal Health

For those who have Barrett's Oesophagus, controlling weight is a complex matter that includes understanding how body weight affects the disease's course as well as the symptoms that accompany it. For this reason, it becomes critical to comprehend the complex relationship between controlling weight and managing Barrett's oesophagus in order to achieve the best possible health and wellbeing. This section seeks to clarify the importance of weight control in relation to Barrett's oesophagus and the possible consequences it may have for those who are managing this illness.

The complex relationship between excess body weight and the escalation of oesophageal symptoms is the foundation of the weight management issue in the context of Barrett's Oesophagus. Several research works have demonstrated a strong correlation between obesity and the exacerbation of gastroesophageal reflux disease (GERD), which is frequently associated with Barrett's oesophagus. Being overweight can put pressure on the stomach, which can push food back up into the oesophagus and result in symptoms like regurgitation and heartburn. Moreover, obesity raises the risk of problems and may accelerate the development of Barrett's oesophagus due to its association with chronic systemic inflammation. Consequently, the task at hand is to tackle the influence of being overweight on the onset and development of Barrett's oesophagus.

There could be a lot of negative effects if the problem of excess body weight is not addressed in the setting of Barrett's Oesophagus. Obesity and Barrett's oesophagus increase the likelihood of severe and recurrent GERD symptoms, which can seriously lower a person's quality of life. The persistent inflammation linked to being overweight can worsen damage to the oesophagus, which may hasten the development of Barrett's oesophagus and raise the risk of dysplasia and cancer. Furthermore, being overweight can make management measures less effective, which makes it more difficult to regulate symptoms connected to Barrett's oesophagus overall.

The adoption of comprehensive weight management measures is the critical strategy to mitigating the effects of excess body weight on Barrett's Oesophagus. Through the implementation of a comprehensive strategy that includes dietary adjustments, physical exercise, and behavioural improvements, individuals can proactively address the detrimental impact of obesity on their gastric health. Adopting these techniques can help create an atmosphere that is favourable for controlling symptoms and managing the illness, which will ultimately lead to better health.

A comprehensive weight-management plan must be implemented using an integrative strategy that includes food changes, exercise, and behavioural changes. Making dietary adjustments could entail switching to a nutrient-dense, well-balanced diet that helps with weight loss and GERD symptom relief. Reducing the intake of high-fat, spicy, and acidic foods while increasing the intake of fruits, vegetables, lean proteins, and whole grains will help minimise GERD symptoms and encourage weight loss. Furthermore, mindful eating techniques and portion control can help with weight management. Physical activity that is customised to each person's skills and interests should be a regular part of weight control and oesophageal health. Moreover, behavioural changes like stress management methods and good sleep hygiene can support food and physical activity interventions in a comprehensive approach to weight management.

Clinical data and research regularly highlight the benefits of weight management for people with Barrett's oesophagus. Research has indicated that making healthy lifestyle changes and losing weight can effectively mitigate symptoms of gastroesophageal reflux disease (GERD) and lessen the intensity of oesophageal inflammation. In addition, people who effectively control their weight report higher overall quality of life and slower Barrett's oesophagus progression.

Following all-inclusive weight-loss plans, patients can expect a significant improvement in their gastric health as well as a reduction in symptoms associated with Barrett's Oesophagus.

Although the main strategy for managing the effects of excess body weight on Barrett's Oesophagus is comprehensive weight control, patients who are severely obese and have GERD symptoms that do not go away may benefit from alternate methods such bariatric surgery. In certain instances, bariatric surgery has proven to be beneficial in encouraging weight loss and reducing GERD symptoms, which may benefit those who have both Barrett's oesophagus and obesity at the same time. But before deciding to have bariatric surgery, a patient should thoroughly assess their medical history and general condition in cooperation with a multidisciplinary healthcare team.

One should not undervalue the importance of maintaining a healthy weight while navigating the challenges of managing Barrett's oesophagus. People can take proactive measures to improve their general well-being, reduce symptoms, and optimise their oesophageal health by adopting complete weight management practises.

Ergonomic Adjustments for Daily Living

This segment's main goal is to give detailed instructions on how to modify everyday activities in an ergonomic way to reduce Barrett's Oesophagus symptoms and improve the general health and quality of life for those who are managing the condition.

It is crucial to have a complete awareness of Barrett's oesophagus, its symptoms, and the potential effects of everyday activities on the condition before starting the process of making ergonomic adjustments in daily living. People will also gain from having access to ergonomic tools and resources that can help them carry out the recommended changes.

In order to reduce discomfort and maximise functionality, making ergonomic changes to one's daily activities and surroundings requires a methodical approach. This procedure involves assessing several aspects of daily living, such as employment, residence, and recreational pursuits, in order to recognise plausible stimuli for esophageal symptoms and putting changes in place to mitigate them.

1. Start by assessing the work environment, taking into account ergonomic elements and workstation configuration. Make sure your desk promotes good posture and less upper-body strain. To ensure ideal alignment and lessen pressure on the oesophagus, adjust the height of the chair, the height of the desk, and the location of the monitor. To create a more comfortable work environment, think about utilising ergonomic devices like ergonomic keyboards, chairs with lumbar support, and adjustable desks.

2. Examine how the kitchen is set up and how meals are prepared to see any possible areas where the oesophagus might be strained. To lessen strain when preparing meals, use countertop heights that minimise bending and reaching and make use of items like long-handled utensils and assistive gadgets. To ensure easy digestion and reduce reflux, concentrate on mindful eating techniques when

dining, such as chewing food well, sitting up straight, and abstaining from hurried or overindulgent eating.

3. Examine the living space to find any areas that might be uncomfortable or stressful. To make moving easier and require less bending, lifting, and reaching, think about optimising the layout and furniture placement. In order to minimise oesophageal pressure and promote good posture, use supportive seating with enough back and arm support.

4. Exercise regimens and physical activities should be adjusted to reduce the possibility of aggravating oesophageal discomfort. Prioritize activities that encourage relaxation and stress reduction, like yoga and light stretching, and go for low-impact workouts that don't put undue strain on the abdomen.

5. To maximise slumber and reduce nocturnal reflux, evaluate the sleeping environment, including the firmness of the mattress, the height of the pillow, and the sleeping position. To raise the upper body as you sleep and lessen the chance of acid reflux, use wedge-shaped pillows or adjustable beds.

- Prioritizing small adjustments and tracking the effects on symptoms over time are essential when implementing ergonomic modifications. Unexpected changes could cause discomfort or resistance.

- Speak with ergonomic specialists or medical professionals to get recommendations that are specific to your requirements and circumstances.

- Strike a balance between rest and exercise, and stay away from repeated motions or extended periods of static posture, which can make oesophageal discomfort worse.

People should keep an eye on their reflux frequency and discomfort levels, as well as monitor their oesophageal symptoms, in order to confirm that the ergonomic improvements have been successfully implemented. Maintain a journal to document how the changes are affecting your everyday activities and general well-being. You can also ask healthcare professionals for their opinions on the changes' effectiveness.

If problems or obstacles arise, people ought to reevaluate the ergonomic changes and think about different strategies. Maintain open lines of contact with your healthcare providers regarding any lingering symptoms or challenges adjusting to the suggested changes.

People with Barrett's oesophagus can improve their comfort and functionality in many areas of their lives and take proactive control of their condition by incorporating these ergonomic changes into their daily lives.

Natural Cleaning and Personal Care Products

When trying to manage Barrett's oesophagus, it's important to take into account environmental elements that can affect one's health in addition to dietary and lifestyle changes. A wide range of chemicals and compounds included in personal care and household cleaning products may worsen symptoms or provide health hazards to those who have Barrett's oesophagus. The purpose of this section is to offer a thorough list of natural substitutes for popular cleaning and personal care products, with an emphasis on how well-suited they are for those who are managing this condition. People can establish a safer and more comfortable living environment that promotes their health and well-being by putting these natural alternatives into practise.

The list that follows offers a carefully chosen range of natural substitutes for popular cleaning and personal care products, each with thorough justifications, supporting data, and useful uses.

a. b. Natural surface cleaners like lemon juice, vinegar, and baking soda are good substitutes for traditional chemical-based cleansers. These organic components have antibacterial qualities and can be used to clean a variety of surfaces, such as appliances, sinks, and counters.

c. Studies have shown that vinegar and lemon juice are efficient natural cleaners because they have antibacterial properties against common home germs. Furthermore, testimonials from people who have Barrett's oesophagus have demonstrated a decrease in cutaneous and respiratory irritation following the use of natural surface cleaners.

d. People can decrease their exposure to harsh chemicals and lower their risk of respiratory irritation and skin sensitivities by include natural surface cleansers in their regular cleaning routines. This will improve indoor air quality.

By lowering potential causes of discomfort and symptoms, switching to natural surface cleaners not only encourages a safer living environment but also fits with the all-encompassing strategy for controlling Barrett's oesophagus.

a. b. Chemical-free laundry detergents offer an alternative to conventional detergents that could include harsh chemicals and perfumes. They are often made with plant-based components and essential oils. These natural detergents lessen the chance of allergic reactions and skin irritation while being kind to the skin.

c. Plant-based laundry detergents have been shown in studies to be less likely to aggravate pre-existing skin issues or trigger skin sensitivities while still being able to remove dirt and stains with effectiveness. Those who have Barrett's oesophagus have attested to the decrease in skin irritation and itching that occurs when they switch to laundry detergents without chemicals.

d. People can reduce skin sensitivity and allergic reactions by using chemical-free laundry detergents, which improves general comfort and well-being while controlling Barrett's oesophagus.

The switch to laundry detergents without chemicals is in line with the overarching objective of lowering chemical exposure and possible discomfort triggers, supporting the treatment of Barrett's oesophagus and enhancing skin health.

a. b. Shampoos, soaps, and lotions made with organic and plant-based ingredients are examples of natural personal care products. They provide a mild and nutritious substitute for traditional products that are packed with harsh chemicals and artificial fragrances. The health of the skin and scalp is the top priority with these natural formulas, which also reduce the chance of irritation and allergic reactions.

c. Studies have shown how natural substances like aloe vera and essential oils can help hydrate skin and reduce inflammation, which supports the usefulness of these compounds in natural personal care products. After switching to natural personal care products, skin and scalp problems improved, according to testimonies from people treating Barrett's oesophagus.

d. People can reduce their risk of allergic responses and skin sensitivities by using natural personal care products in their regular hygiene routines. This will promote general skin health and comfort while controlling Barrett's oesophagus.

Using natural personal care products can help enhance quality of life and well-being by addressing potential triggers for skin sensitivities and allergic reactions, which is in line with the holistic approach to controlling Barrett's oesophagus.

a. b Natural essential oil diffusers and handmade room sprays are examples of non-toxic air fresheners that offer an alternative to traditional air fresheners that contain volatile organic compounds and artificial aromas (VOCs). These natural substitutes for chemical-based air fresheners offer pleasing scents without the risk of irritating the respiratory system.

c. Studies have shown that natural essential oils may have respiratory advantages, such as the capacity to ease stress and encourage relaxation, which supports the usage of these oils in non-toxic air fresheners. Patients with Barrett's oesophagus have reported decreased headaches and respiratory pain following the switch to non-toxic air fresheners.

d. Research has demonstrated the potential respiratory advantages of natural essential oils, such as their capacity to ease stress and encourage relaxation, which supports their usage in safe air fresheners. Reportedly, switching to non-toxic air fresheners reduced headaches and discomfort in the respiratory system among those with Barrett's oesophagus.

The Future of Barrett's Oesophagus Treatment

Innovative Research and Clinical Trials

Introduction to the Topic:

Due to its propensity to develop to esophageal cancer, Barrett's Esophagus—a disorder marked by the change of the normal squamous epithelium of the oesophagus into columnar epithelium—is a serious issue. Innovative studies and clinical trials have been carried out over time to learn more about this illness and create efficient treatment plans. The purpose of this chapter is to provide an overview of the state of Barrett's oesophagus research and clinical trials, as well as any prospective management implications.

This chapter will investigate the assertion that continued research and clinical trials are essential to improving our knowledge of Barrett's oesophagus and creating more efficient treatment plans.

The increasing amount of research on the molecular mechanisms behind the onset and progression of Barrett's oesophagus is one of the main pieces of evidence in favour of the claim. Research has shown particular genetic and epigenetic changes linked to the development of esophageal adenocarcinoma from Barrett's oesophagus, offering important new targets for therapeutic intervention.

Delve Deeper into the Evidence:

A closer look at this data shows that the discovery of important molecular pathways connected to the pathophysiology of Barrett's oesophagus has made focused treatment development possible. Preclinical models and early-phase clinical studies have demonstrated encouraging outcomes in clinical trials examining the effectiveness of molecularly targeted medicines, such as inhibitors of particular signalling pathways implicated in the evolution of Barrett's oesophagus.

It is crucial to recognise that although targeted therapies have promise, creating treatments that are universally effective will be difficult due to the heterogeneity of Barrett's oesophagus and the intricate interactions between hereditary and environmental factors. Furthermore, problems with drug resistance and off-target effects have been reported in several clinical trials assessing targeted medicines, underscoring the need for more development and individualised strategies.

In answer to the counterarguments, it is critical to stress that, despite obstacles, current research in biomarker identification and precision medicine strives to find patient-specific traits that can guide treatment choices and enhance therapeutic outcomes. Furthermore, the amalgamation of multi-omics data, encompassing transcriptomics, proteomics, and genomes, exhibits potential in deciphering the molecular intricacies of Barrett's Esophagus and steering the creation of more customised therapies.

Apart from targeted medicines, immunotherapeutic techniques have gained significance in the treatment of esophageal cancer and Barrett's oesophagus. Clinical trials examining adoptive cell treatments and immune checkpoint inhibitors have shown promising outcomes in a minority of patients, highlighting the potential for immunotherapy to supplement current treatment approaches. Establish expectations for the reader by providing a concise and well-structured list of the terms that need to be defined.

To sum up, the data demonstrates how important it is for new research and clinical studies to advance our knowledge of Barrett's oesophagus and its care. The continuous search of tailored treatments, immunotherapeutic approaches, and precision medicine holds promise for enhancing patient outcomes and lessening the burden of chronic illness, despite obstacles and difficulties. Researchers, physicians, and patients must work together to advance the development of more efficient care strategies as we learn more about the complexities of Barrett's oesophagus.

Advancements in Diagnostic Technology

Early discovery of Barrett's oesophagus can have a substantial impact on patient outcomes, making diagnosis a crucial part of treatment. Histopathological analysis of biopsy samples and endoscopic assessment have historically been the mainstays of the diagnosis. On the other hand, improvements in diagnostic technologies may improve Barrett's Esophagus diagnosis accessibility, effectiveness, and accuracy, leading to better patient outcomes.

The main problem in diagnosing Barrett's oesophagus is that traditional diagnostic techniques like endoscopy and histopathology have drawbacks, such as the possibility of sampling errors and inter-observer variability. These restrictions may result in inadequate monitoring plans, delayed diagnosis of dysplasia or early-stage neoplasia, and missed diagnoses, all of which may have an adverse effect on patient outcomes.

Patients with Barrett's oesophagus may be at danger of undiagnosed disease progression, or esophageal cancer, if the issue of inadequate diagnostic accuracy is not appropriately addressed. In addition, insufficient and consistent diagnostic techniques may lead to needless monitoring measures, patient distress, and inefficiencies in the use of healthcare resources.

Barrett's oesophagus diagnosis can be made more accurately and precisely by integrating molecular biomarkers, artificial intelligence (AI) technology, and modern imaging modalities. This approach addresses the shortcomings of existing diagnostic techniques.

Barrett's Esophagus mucosal and submucosal alterations can be better seen with the use of modern imaging modalities such confocal laser endomicroscopy (CLE), narrow-band imaging (NBI), and high-definition endoscopy. With the use of these technologies, tissue architecture and vasculature may be characterised in real time, which can help identify dysplastic and neoplastic lesions with greater sensitivity and specificity.

Moreover, the integration of molecular biomarkers, such as protein biomarkers, gene expression profiles, and DNA methylation markers, into diagnostic algorithms may improve the precision of the diagnosis of Barrett's oesophagus. In the end, these biomarkers can enable individualised treatment plans by offering more details on the course of the disease, risk assessment, and therapeutic response prediction.

Another crucial component of the solution is the use of AI-based technologies for pattern identification and image analysis. Barrett's oesophagus and related neoplasia can be automatically detected and classified with the help of machine learning algorithms that have been trained on massive datasets of endoscopic pictures and histopathological samples. This could lower inter-observer variability and enhance diagnostic consistency.

Research assessing the application of molecular biomarkers, artificial intelligence, and sophisticated imaging modalities in Barrett's esophageal reflux disease diagnosis have shown encouraging results. With the increased diagnosis accuracy for dysplastic and neoplastic alterations brought about by advanced imaging techniques, high-risk patients can now benefit from tailored therapy and improved surveillance.

Furthermore, the integration of molecular biomarkers into diagnostic algorithms has demonstrated the ability to classify individuals according to their likelihood of developing a disease and to inform individualised surveillance and treatment choices. AI-based technologies have proven to be able to help endoscopists anticipate the histological categorization of Barrett's oesophagus and identify small abnormalities of the mucosa, thus improving the consistency and confidence of diagnosis.

While combining molecular biomarkers, artificial intelligence, and advanced imaging modalities offers a promising way to improve the diagnosis of Barrett's oesophagus, it's important to recognise that there are other options as well, like non-endoscopic screening modalities and the creation of minimally invasive or non-invasive diagnostic tests. Particularly for surveillance in high-risk populations, non-endoscopic methods like capsule endoscopy and transnasal endoscopy may be more patient-friendly and accessible. Moreover, a developing field of study that has the potential to completely transform diagnostic approaches in the future is the investigation of blood-based biomarkers and exhaled breath analysis for the non-invasive identification of Barrett's oesophagus and related neoplasia.

To sum up, the amalgamation of sophisticated imaging modalities, molecular biomarkers, and artificial intelligence technologies exhibits considerable potential in surmounting the constraints of conventional diagnostic techniques for Barrett's oesophagus. The potential for these developments to be implemented could lead to improved patient outcomes and the efficient management of this ailment by improving risk classification, individualised management, and diagnostic accuracy. The advancement of diagnostic technology in Barrett's Esophagus has the potential to revolutionise clinical practise and improve patient care as long as continuous research keeps advancing and validating these diagnostic techniques.

Genetic Research and Personalized Medicine

Our understanding of Barrett's oesophagus has been completely transformed by genetic research, which has opened new avenues for personalised treatment methods and provided insights into the underlying molecular pathways. Researchers have found promising biomarkers, therapeutic targets, and prognostic indicators that hold great promise for customised care regimens by identifying the genetic determinants of this disorder. This chapter explores the relationship between personalised medicine and genetic research in the context of Barrett's oesophagus, and how genetic discoveries may affect future developments in diagnosis, prognosis, and treatment.

The potential for improving patient outcomes and prognosis through personalised medicine treatments for Barrett's oesophagus through the integration of genetic research discoveries into clinical practise is significant.

Finding genetic variations linked to the development and susceptibility of Barrett's oesophagus is one of the main goals of genetic research on the condition. Genetic loci that provide an elevated risk of Barrett's oesophagus and its development to esophageal cancer have been identified by genome-wide association studies (GWAS). For example, the pathophysiology of Barrett's Esophagus has been linked to single nucleotide polymorphisms (SNPs) in genes involved in the inflammatory response, cell proliferation, and DNA repair pathways, providing insight into the condition's molecular causes.

Moreover, the clarification of somatic genetic changes in the development of esophageal adenocarcinoma from Barrett's oesophagus has yielded significant information about the molecular progression of this illness. Genetic abnormalities that drive malignant transformation have been identified in studies describing the landscape of somatic mutations, copy number changes, and chromosomal rearrangements in Barrett's Esophagus-associated neoplasia. These findings provide potential targets for precision therapies and prognostic markers for the progression of the disease.

The discovery of genetic variations linked to susceptibility to Barrett's esophagitis not only advances our knowledge of the disease's aetiology but also has implications for risk assessment and customised screening procedures. Clinicians can identify patients who are at a higher risk of acquiring Barrett's oesophagus by incorporating genetic risk scores obtained from susceptibility loci. This allows for targeted surveillance and early intervention techniques to slow the progression of the disease.

Furthermore, the identification of somatic genetic changes in Barrett's esophagus-associated neoplasia may help develop focused treatment strategies. Targeted therapies and immunotherapies that are customised to the molecular profile of each patient's tumour can be used in personalised therapy regimens made possible by the detection of actionable genetic abnormalities, such as mutations in tumour suppressor genes or oncogenes.

Although incorporating genetic research into customised care for Barrett's oesophagus holds great potential, there are obstacles in converting genomic discoveries into clinical applications. The intricacy of genetic relationships and the polygenic nature of illness susceptibility are one such difficulty. The combination of several genetic variants, each enumerating a little risk, makes it difficult to reliably estimate an individual's risk of a disease based alone on genetic markers.

Additionally, the availability of targeted agents and the viability of integrating molecularly guided treatment paradigms into standard clinical care are prerequisites for the clinical utility of somatic genetic alterations as practicable targets for therapy in Barrett's Esophagus-associated neoplasia.

In order to improve the accuracy of risk prediction models, it is necessary to integrate genetic risk scores with other risk factors, such as environmental exposures, lifestyle factors, and clinical parameters, in order to address the complexity of polygenic disease susceptibility and its translation to clinical practise. The arsenal of targeted therapies is also growing as a result of continued work in pharmacogenomics and medication development, which presents the possibility of customised treatment plans based on the molecular characteristics of certain tumours.

Barrett's oesophagus has additional genetic complexity due to epigenetic modifications, such as DNA methylation patterns and histone modifications, in addition to genetic variations and somatic mutations. The course of disease is significantly influenced by epigenetic dysregulation, which presents prospective biomarkers for risk assessment and treatment targets. Knowing how genetic and epigenetic changes interact offers a thorough basis for personalised medicine approaches to Barrett's oesophagus care.

To sum up, the incorporation of genetic research results into personalised medicine techniques for Barrett's oesophagus has great potential to improve the accuracy and effectiveness of prognostic, therapeutic, and diagnostic methods. Clinicians can improve patient outcomes and prognosis by customising monitoring, screening, and therapy plans for each patient by utilising genetic information. Personalized medicine in the management of Barrett's oesophagus is about to become a reality thanks to continued breakthroughs in genetic and genomic technology and interdisciplinary collaborations. However, there are still hurdles in transferring genetic research into clinical practise.

The Role of Artificial Intelligence in Treatment

Over the years, artificial intelligence (AI) has been a disruptive force in the healthcare industry, changing the paradigms of diagnosis and treatment. The potential role of AI in assisting with diagnosis and management holds great promise in the setting of Barrett's Esophagus, where prompt and precise diagnosis is crucial. In order to shed light on the opportunities and difficulties involved in utilising AI for improved patient care, this chapter aims to investigate how AI technologies can be integrated into the overall management of Barrett's oesophagus.

The current state of Barrett's esophagitis diagnosis is marked by difficulties in obtaining high levels of efficiency and accuracy in risk assessment and disease identification. While essential to the therapy of Barrett's oesophagus, traditional endoscopic surveillance and histological assessment are mostly dependent on visual interpretation and are vulnerable to interobserver variability, which may result in incorrect risk categorization or missed diagnoses. Furthermore, in order to promote early intervention and enhance patient outcomes, scalable and precise diagnostic techniques are required due to the rising incidence of Barrett's oesophagus and the neoplasia that it is associated with.

There are several consequences associated with inadequate or postponed diagnosis of Barrett's oesophagus. First off, a patient's prognosis and longevity may be greatly impacted by the condition's progression from underlying dysplasia to invasive adenocarcinoma due to missed or delayed discovery. Second, inequalities in illness identification and risk stratification across healthcare settings are caused by clinical practise variability, which is a result of the absence of standardised and scalable diagnostic techniques. Patients may thus encounter a delay in receiving necessary interventions, which could negatively affect their general quality of life and medical results.

The difficulties in diagnosing and treating Barrett's oesophagus can be effectively overcome by integrating AI-powered tools and algorithms. AI technologies, such as deep learning and machine learning algorithms, have the potential to improve prognostication, risk assessment, and illness detection accuracy and efficiency. This will provide doctors with useful information for individualised patient care.

The use of AI in the context of Barrett's Esophagus entails the creation and verification of AI models that have been trained on a variety of datasets, including clinical data, histological specimens, and endoscopic images. These artificial intelligence (AI) models can be created to automatically detect and describe Barrett's oesophagus, differentiate dysplastic lesions, and forecast the course of the disease. They can also be used to enhance clinical decision-making by utilising pattern recognition and data-driven insights.

Additionally, real-time support for endoscopists through automated lesion diagnosis and enhanced visualisation is made possible by the integration of AI technologies into endoscopic imaging platforms. This improves the accuracy and efficiency of endoscopic surveillance for Barrett's oesophagus.

Research on the use of AI in Barrett's oesophagus has produced encouraging results. In certain cases, AI algorithms have outperformed human interpreters in terms of sensitivity and specificity when it comes to diagnosing Barrett's oesophagus and dysplastic alterations. AI integration in endoscopic settings has also demonstrated promise in decreasing missed lesions and raising the overall diagnostic yield of endoscopic surveillance, which could improve the timeliness and precision of disease diagnosis.

Barrett's oesophagus management through AI integration has a lot of potential, but in order to fully utilise the capabilities of AI technologies, complementary strategies like the creation of standardised protocols for endoscopic surveillance and histopathological assessment must be taken into account. The optimal use of AI in clinical practise is contingent upon interdisciplinary cooperation and the harmonisation of AI with established clinical workflows, since this ensures seamless integration and optimal utility.

In summary, the prospective application of AI to the diagnosis and treatment of Barrett's oesophagus signifies a paradigm shift in the all-encompassing care of this illness. In the era of Barrett's oesophagus management, doctors can improve patient outcomes and customised medicine methods by utilising AI technology to improve the accuracy, efficiency, and scalability of disease diagnosis and risk assessment.

New research demonstrates how AI can help with disease detection, disease trajectory prediction, and treatment response prediction. The potential for personalised prognostication and therapeutic stratification is presented by AI-driven predictive models that incorporate multi-modal data, such as genetic, imaging, and clinical parameters. This paves the way for precision medicine and tailored interventions in the management of Barrett's oesophagus.

A new era of precision and personalised medicine is being ushered in by the integration of AI into the management of Barrett's oesophagus. This technology has the potential to revolutionise diagnostic and therapeutic paradigms and ultimately improve patient care and outcomes in the management of this challenging condition. Even though there are obstacles in the way of the smooth integration and validation of AI technologies, continued progress and joint efforts are well-positioned to propel the realisation of AI-enhanced precision medicine in the overall care of Barrett's oesophagus.

Preventive Strategies and Screening

The hallmark of Barrett's Esophagus is the metaplastic columnar epithelium that develops in the oesophagus in response to persistent gastroesophageal reflux illness, replacing the normal squamous epithelium (GERD). People who have this metaplastic alteration are more likely to develop esophageal adenocarcinoma, a cancer that has a poor prognosis and few therapeutic options when discovered at an advanced stage. Preventive methods and screening are important in managing Barrett's oesophagus because they can help identify individuals who are at high risk, make early intervention easier, and eventually lessen the burden of esophageal adenocarcinoma.

Variability in clinical practise and inequities in disease diagnosis are caused by the lack of globally agreed standards for population-based screening and preventative measures, despite advances in our understanding of Barrett's oesophagus and its progression to adenocarcinoma. This lack of uniformity makes it difficult to identify people who are at-risk, put in place suitable surveillance systems, and put preventive measures in place to lessen the chance that esophageal adenocarcinoma will develop.

The lack of organised preventative measures and screening procedures for Barrett's oesophagus has real-world ramifications that affect individuals as well as the general public. Individually, failing to recognise and keep an eye on high-risk patients may lead to missed opportunities for prompt care, which could progress Barrett's oesophagus to advanced neoplasia and have a negative impact on patient morbidity and death. From a public health standpoint, the lack of efficacious screening methods contributes to the societal burden of esophageal adenocarcinoma by increasing its influence on patient outcomes and the use of healthcare resources.

One key way to overcome the difficulties in managing Barrett's oesophagus is to develop evidence-based guidelines for risk assessment, population-based screening, and customised preventative measures. These recommendations ought to cover risk factor evaluation, endoscopic surveillance procedures, and the application of preventative strategies, such pharmacological therapies and lifestyle adjustments, in populations of individuals who are at risk.

The successful execution of screening protocols and preventative measures requires a multidisciplinary approach combining the cooperation of public health organisations, primary care physicians, and gastroenterologists. Tools for risk stratification that combine endoscopic, clinical, and demographic data can help identify people who are more likely to develop Barrett's oesophagus and direct the deployment of monitoring resources. Furthermore, early diagnosis of dysplastic alterations and neoplastic progression can be facilitated by the adoption of defined endoscopic surveillance intervals, guided by risk classification. This allows for timely intervention and customised care.

Adoption of population-based screening and preventative measures has been shown to improve outcomes for a number of cancers, such as cervical and colorectal cancer. Applying these achievements to the Barrett's Esophagus setting, it is anticipated that systematic screening and preventative care will improve the early identification of esophageal adenocarcinoma and high-grade dysplasia, slowing the advancement of the illness and enhancing patient outcomes.

Apart from population-based screening, alternative methods offer supplementary strategies to enhance the efficacy of preventive interventions. These methods include the identification of molecular biomarkers for risk stratification and the investigation of non-invasive diagnostic modalities, such as imaging techniques and biomarker-based tests. These non-invasive options have the potential to improve the accuracy and scalability of disease diagnosis and risk assessment when combined with traditional endoscopic surveillance, supporting all-encompassing Barrett's esophageal therapy.

To sum up, the incorporation of screening protocols and preventive techniques is a crucial aspect of managing Barrett's oesophagus comprehensively. This approach has the ability to lessen the severity of esophageal cancer and enhance patient outcomes. Through the development of evidence-based protocols and the implementation of systematic risk assessment and surveillance, medical professionals can proactively detect high-risk patients, promptly initiate interventions, and ultimately propel the field of precision medicine forward in the treatment of Barrett's oesophagus.

New research highlights how non-invasive screening techniques, like molecular biomarker panels and capsule endoscopy, can help with risk stratification and early Barrett's esophagitis identification. When incorporated into screening algorithms, these modalities hold the potential to improve population-based screening's acceptability and scalability, which could ultimately lower the burden of esophageal cancer.

An era of proactive and individualised care for Barrett's oesophagus is being ushered in with the adoption of evidence-based preventive methods and screening protocols. Clinicians can optimise patient care and results in the management of this complicated condition by utilising risk stratification techniques, organised monitoring intervals, and supplementary screening modalities. These strategies can help to increase the precision and scalability of disease diagnosis. Although there remain obstacles in the way of integrating and validating these strategies, further progress and joint efforts hold promise for bringing about a proactive and preventative paradigm in the care of Barrett's oesophagus.

Patient Advocacy and Policy Change

In order to improve treatment access and drive policy change for people with Barrett's oesophagus, patient advocacy is essential. Advocacy initiatives can impact regulatory decisions, advance fair access to care, and spark revolutionary changes in healthcare policies by defending the rights and needs of patients. In the context of Barrett's Esophagus, this chapter explores the importance of patient advocacy, describing the obstacles, repercussions of inaction, suggested remedies, and possible results of changing policy as a result of advocacy activities.

Precancerous Barrett's oesophagus, which is caused by chronic gastroesophageal reflux disease, is a serious health risk since it is linked to esophageal adenocarcinoma, a cancer that has a high risk of morbidity and mortality. The need for comprehensive policy reforms to address the unmet needs of afflicted individuals is underscored by the persistence of gaps in access to screening, surveillance, and preventative measures despite the increased prevalence of Barrett's oesophagus. In light of this, patient advocacy becomes clear as a powerful tool for bringing about change by elevating the voices of persons affected by Barrett's oesophagus and promoting laws that give priority to early detection, individualised treatment, and better results.

The main problem at hand is that there are differences in the availability of prompt screening, surveillance, and successful interventions for people with Barrett's oesophagus due to the absence of standardised policies and insufficient support. This discrepancy makes it more difficult to detect high-risk patients early on and to put preventive measures in place that could slow the condition's progression to esophageal cancer. In addition, the lack of strong policies makes impacted people feel more alone and makes it harder for them to navigate the complicated healthcare system on their own with little help or resources.

The effects of inaction are complex and include both social and personal repercussions. Individuals with Barrett's oesophagus may experience delayed diagnosis, restricted access to specialised care, and possibly worse health outcomes as a result of a lack of policy-driven support. Moreover, the lack of all-encompassing policies exacerbates inequality, increasing discrepancies in healthcare accessibility and prolonging the illness burden among susceptible groups. The therapy of advanced esophageal adenocarcinoma has significant social and economic expenses in addition to jeopardising the well-being of affected persons.

Promoting legislative changes that give fair access to screening, monitoring, and preventive care for people with Barrett's oesophagus top priority is the way to find a solution. This entails using the combined clout of patient advocacy groups to work with legislators, healthcare providers, and other pertinent parties to create and carry out laws that meet the unmet needs of those who are impacted. Furthermore, it is imperative to develop evidence-based guidelines that are influenced by clinical knowledge and patient views in order to effectively drive policy changes that contribute to improving outcomes and lowering the incidence of esophageal adenocarcinoma.

A deliberate and cooperative strategy is required for the implementation of policy changes, requiring the active participation of patient advocacy groups, healthcare providers, researchers, and lawmakers. Establishing thorough screening programmes, standardising surveillance procedures, and incorporating patient-centered care models into legislative frameworks ought to be the top priorities of this partnership. Furthermore, it is essential to include patient-reported outcomes and lived experiences in policy debates to make sure that the suggested changes are in line with the objectives and requirements of those who are impacted by Barrett's oesophagus.

In the past, legislative reforms motivated by lobbying have produced revolutionary results in the healthcare industry by promoting better access to care, increased financing for research, and the prioritisation of patient-centered programmes. Extrapolating these accomplishments to the Barrett's Esophagus setting, higher clinical outcomes for those at risk of esophageal adenocarcinoma are anticipated as a result of patient advocacy-driven policy changes that increase awareness and streamline care pathways. Furthermore, these policy adjustments may promote a more welcoming and encouraging healthcare environment that gives people with Barrett's oesophagus the ability to actively engage in their treatment and decision-making.

The expansion of community-based support programmes, the encouragement of health literacy initiatives, and the establishment of peer-to-peer support networks are some alternative strategies that can be used in addition to the primary solution of advocating for policy changes to address the complex needs of people with Barrett's oesophagus. These substitutes not only strengthen the effects of lobbying-driven legislation modifications, but they also highlight the all-encompassing strategy required for proper Barrett's oesophagus care.

In summary, patient advocacy can be a driving force behind changes in legislation and can enhance treatment accessibility for those who have Barrett's oesophagus. Patient advocacy groups can effect transformative changes that resonate across healthcare systems, ultimately improving the quality of life and prognosis for individuals affected by this complex condition by advocating for equitable policies that prioritise early detection, personalised care, and improved outcomes. Thus, a more inclusive and patient-centered paradigm for Barrett's oesophagus management could be shaped by the cooperation of patient advocates, healthcare stakeholders, and legislators.

Hope on the Horizon: Promising Developments

The Barrett's Esophagus Mastery Bible is your all-inclusive road map for navigating and becoming an expert in Barrett's Esophagus management—not it's just another medical guide. Your relationship with Barrett's oesophagus will change as a result of the priceless insights, empowering techniques, and profound grasp of holistic healthcare that you will acquire on this life-changing trip. With the help of this book, you should be able to take control of your health, regain your wellbeing, and look forward to a future devoid of anxiety and uncertainty.

The approaches described in this guide are not only theories; rather, they are founded in years of clinical experience, evidence-based procedures, and a thorough comprehension of the complex characteristics of Barrett's oesophagus. I, Dr. Ankita Kashyap, along with my interdisciplinary team of specialists from many health and wellness domains have painstakingly assembled an abundance of knowledge including lifestyle adjustments, customised meal plans, mental health counselling, self-care methods, and coping mechanisms. When included into your daily routine, these techniques serve as the cornerstone of a comprehensive and long-term strategy for controlling Barrett's oesophagus, building resilience, and improving your general state of health.

It is normal to be sceptical when presented with the intricacies of a long-term illness like Barrett's oesophagus. But don't worry—none of the information in this book is predicated on spurious claims or easy fixes. Instead, it is based on the combination of clinical knowledge, scientific study, and firsthand accounts from people who have successfully overcome the difficulties associated with Barrett's oesophagus. Through the adoption of a patient-centered and holistic strategy, we tackle scepticism head-on, demolishing it with an abundance of tried-and-true methods and enlightening perspectives intended to give you hope and confidence as you pursue maximum health.

Imagine a life in which Barrett's Esophagus is not a burden that limits your options or jeopardises your health. Imagine yourself in the future, equipped with the information and resources you need to take charge of your health, live a vibrant life, and confidently take on new challenges. This book's transforming journey is about encouraging a deep change in your connection with your Barrett's oesophagus so that you can take back control of your health and well-being, not merely about controlling symptoms. If you put the holistic solutions into practise, you will see a transformation that goes beyond simple management and results in a life that is resilient and full of life.

This book's material is valuable in ways that go much beyond conventional medical advice. It goes beyond that and encompasses resilience, empowerment, and the possibility of radical life change. Adhering to the ideas and tactics presented in these pages is more than simply starting a learning trip; it means choosing a route that leads to complete health, energy, and a future free from Barrett's Esophagus' constraints. This is a commitment to more than just the book—a it's commitment to your well-being, your own future, and the possibility that you will one day become an expert on Barrett's Esophagus.

In my capacity as the author, "Dr. Ankita Kashyap," I fervently support holistic medicine and wellbeing. This transforming guide is the result of my passion for enabling people to overcome the limitations imposed by chronic diseases, in conjunction with my clinical experience and dedication to evidence-based approaches. I'm committed to giving you the skills, information, and encouragement you need to start a journey toward holistic health and well-being that goes beyond the constraints frequently connected to long-term illnesses, together with my team of professionals.

By combining food plans tailored to your needs, psychological counselling, self-care methods, and coping mechanisms, this book aims to provide you with a thorough framework covering the psychological, emotional, and physical aspects of managing Barrett's oesophagus. It is a testimonial to the ability of holistic treatment to change lives and promote resilience in the face of chronic conditions, not just a manual.

As you read through "The Barrett's Esophagus Mastery Bible," picture a time when the complexities of Barrett's Esophagus don't cloud your life; instead, they will serve as a driving force behind your resilience, personal development, and empowered well-being. This is more than just a book—your it's road map to taking back authority, loving life, and negotiating Barrett's Esophagus's complexity with a fresh feeling of empowerment and hope.

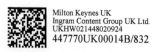